Chicken Soup for the Soul®

Inspiration for Nurses

Chicken Soup for the Soul: Inspiration for Nurses
101 Stories of Appreciation & Wisdom
Amy Newmark, LeAnn Thieman.

Published by Chicken Soup for the Soul Publishing, LLC www.chickensoup.com

The publisher gratefully acknowledges the many publishers and individuals who granted Chicken Soup for the Soul permission to reprint the cited material.

Front cover photo courtesy of iStockphoto.com/MKurtbas (© Mutlu Kurtbas).
Back cover and interior photo courtesy of iStockphoto.com/Ranplett (© Ranplett).
Photo of Amy Newmark courtesy of Susan Morrow at SwickPix.

Cover Design by Brian Taylor, Pneuma Books, LLC
Layout by Marie Killoran

Distributed to the booktrade by Simon & Schuster. SAN: 200-2442

Publisher's Cataloging-In-Publication Data
(Prepared by The Donohue Group, Inc.)

Chicken soup for the soul : inspiration for nurses : 101 stories of appreciation & wisdom / [compiled by] Amy Newmark [and] LeAnn Thieman.

pages ; cm

ISBN: 978-1-61159-948-0

1. Nurses--Literary collections. 2. Nurses--Anecdotes. 3. Nursing--Literary collections. 4. Nursing--Anecdotes. 5. Anecdotes. I. Newmark, Amy. II. Thieman, LeAnn. III. Title: Inspiration for nurses : 101 stories of appreciation & wisdom

RT61 .C45 2015
610.73/02 2015938137

PRINTED IN THE UNITED STATES OF AMERICA
on acid∞free paper

23 22 21 08 09 10 11

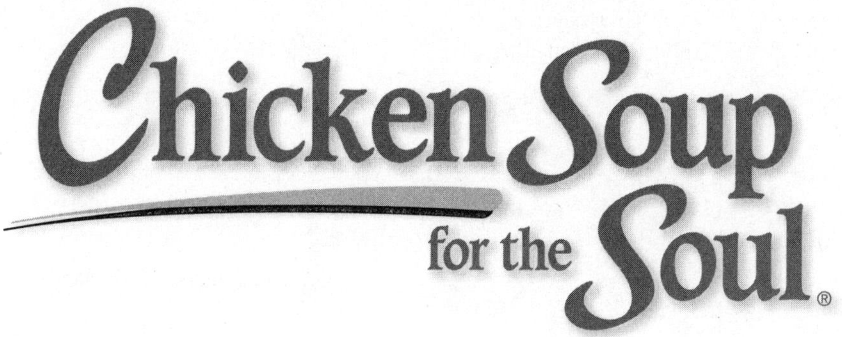

Inspiration for Nurses

101 Stories of Appreciation & Wisdom

Amy Newmark
LeAnn Thieman

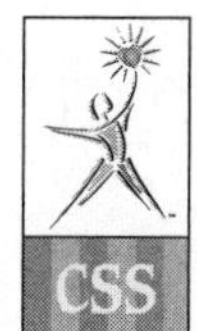

Chicken Soup for the Soul Publishing, LLC
Cos Cob, CT

Chicken Soup for the Soul®

For moments that become stories™

www.chickensoup.com

To all the nurses who,
perhaps more than any other group on Earth,
truly ease the suffering in the world.

Contents

6

~Divine Intervention~

7

~Angels Among Us~

8

~A Matter of Perspective~

9

~Beyond the Call of Duty~

10

~Heart of a Nurse~

11
~Thank You~

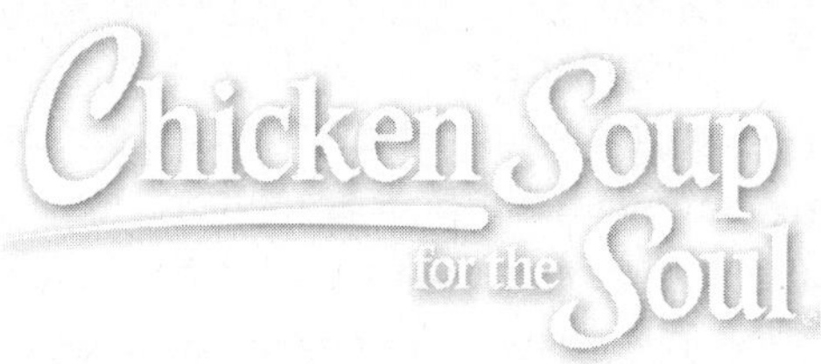

Introduction

Well, my beloved colleagues, we did it again!

I'm often asked which book is better, the original edition of *Chicken Soup for the Nurse's Soul*, or the *Second Dose* edition. I always boast that, because of the thousands of amazing stories submitted by nurses, they are equally fantastic. And now, for a third time, you sent us stories that exceeded every expectation!

You shared true stories from pediatrics (we learn so much from kids in stories like "A Measure of Love") to geriatrics (yes, you can have snowball fights in nursing homes as proven in "Confession of a Nurse"). From caring for newborn babies ("Angels in the NICU") to troubled teens ("The Invulnerable Child") to end-of-life care for the elderly ("In the Sweet By and By"), these stories reveal our tender ministrations throughout the cycles of life.

There are stories for every nurse, regardless of age, gender, experience, or expertise. Nurses offered their stories from almost every field, including schools, missions, volunteering, float, long-term care, transplants, OR, emergency, home health, students, instructors, new grads, psych, sexual assault, holistic, hospice, and more.

Incredibly, we received some from almost every family member. Children wrote about discovering the importance of their moms' work in "The Bus Stop" and "What Does Your Mom Do?" A husband shared poignant revelations in "The Spouse of a Nurse."

You'll laugh yourself silly when you read "Inappropriate" and wipe tears of pride as you relate to the grateful emotions shared by a mother in "You Were My Arms."

The breadth of what we do is beautifully demonstrated in these pages, recounting how we heal bodies ("Nurse Jesse"), minds ("The Gold Miners"), and spirits of our patients ("A Nurse Named Michael").

You'll enjoy an entire chapter on angels, proving that nurses truly are angels of mercy. Another chapter shares incidents that most people believed were Beyond the Call of Duty, even though the nurses thought they were simply doing their jobs... on duty or off. Whether a simple bath ("A Better Nurse") or backrub ("Keeping the Pace") or intensive care ("Privileged Presence"), our hands and hearts bring healing.

These days, things seem to be getting harder and harder in health care, and staying positive and motivated can be a real challenge. In this book you will find inspiration to keep on caring. The entire last chapter is a Thank You, to all of you who give so selflessly.

So keep a well-worn copy in your locker, backpack, nurse's station, bathroom or break room. Read stories in solitude or together as a team. You'll be reminded why we entered this profession... and why we stay.

This book is not only our gift to you, it is your gift to one another. We hope it brings you all of the hope, health and healing you bring to those you serve.

For every hand you've held, song you have sung, and life you have touched, we thank you with all our hearts.

~LeAnn Thieman

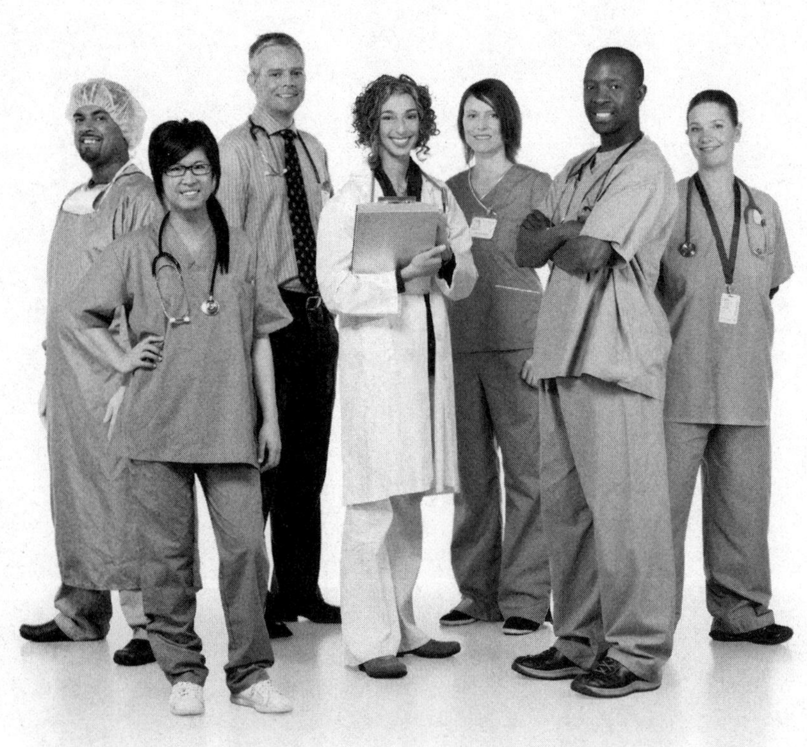

Inspiration for Nurses

The True Meaning of Nursing

Constant attention by a good nurse may be just as important as a major operation by a surgeon.

~Dag Hammarskjöld

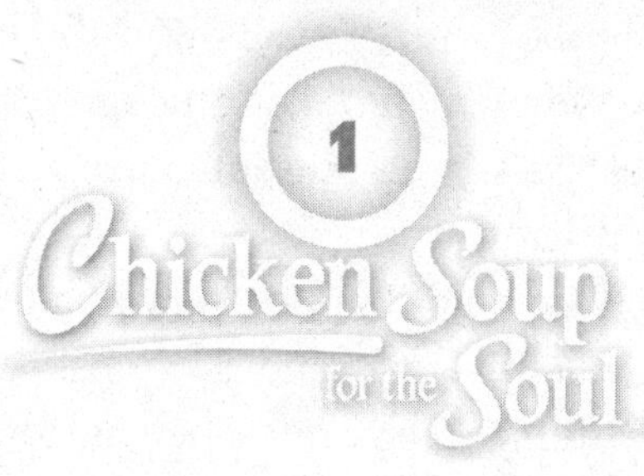

Twelve-Hour Talks

When the whole world is silent,
even one voice becomes powerful.
~Malala Yousafzai

John and I spent several weeks of twelve-hour night shifts together. He lay motionless and unresponsive, connected to IV fluids, a feeding tube, and a Foley catheter. As a registered nurse in a neuro-trauma intensive care unit, I cared for this twenty-something patient, comatose after a car crash. Although his other injuries were minor, his brain was jostled. Day shift reported that his mother visited each morning, but he had no company except for me from 7:00 p.m. until 7:00 a.m.

As much for myself as for John, I kept up a running conversation each time I entered his room. "Good evening John, this is Saturday." "It's cold and cloudy outside. Do you like rain?" It didn't matter to me that John did not answer. I continued our conversations as though he had. When the television was on I discussed the program and the news of the day. When I bathed him and changed his linens I discussed the pros and cons of baths versus showers. If the traffic was bad on my way to work, I told him about it, along with running discussions about everything from sports to cafeteria food. When it was time for my day off, I told him what I would be doing and when I would return. John never responded but I talked anyway.

One evening, when I returned from several days off, John was not in his room. Fearing the worst, I swallowed the lump in my throat and focused on my new patients. I'd long ago learned that nursing is a job where crises are shared but outcomes aren't always known. Sometimes it's better that way.

Weeks went by. One night I noticed a woman walking in the hall beside a tall young man using a cane. They paused at each room as if listening for something. "They must be someone's family in for a visit," I told myself, as I watched their slow progress. I gathered the supplies I needed from the nurse's station and started to my patient's room when another nurse stepped into the hall and asked me a question. As I answered her, the young man's head turned. He quickened his pace and approached me. "I know your voice."

"Can I help you?"

"You already did," he laughed.

"John! I didn't recognize you standing upright and dressed in jeans and a T-shirt!"

His mother explained that he had regained consciousness and had been moved to a rehab floor, where he made rapid progress.

"He did not remember his accident, but did remember a voice during his time in the 'twilight,' as he called it. At first I dismissed it as a dream or his imagination, but John insisted it was real," his mother explained.

John explained: "So I had Mom bring me to this unit, first on day shift and then again on evening shift, so I could listen for the voice. Your voice: the voice that calmed my fears and brought me comfort."

John's smile and hug reminded me why, for twenty years, I have been a nurse.

~Sharon T. Hinton

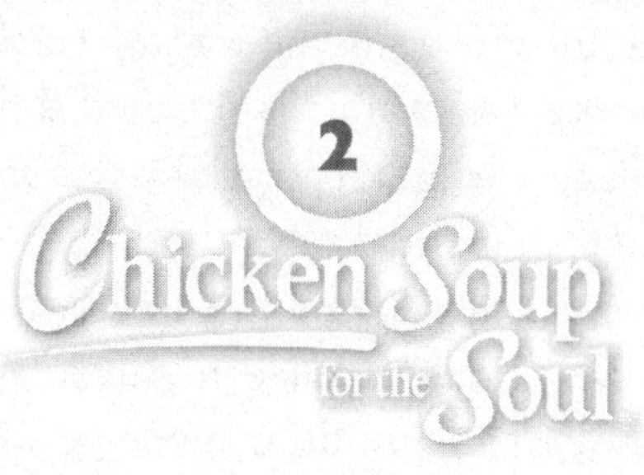

Above and Beyond

Hope is life and life is hope.
~Adele Shreve

Kevin was tethered to machines that clicked and blinked and beeped. His normal exuberance diminished as he was kept immobile. We, his family, knew his humor was still intact, but weakness was sapping it away.

So many nurses, therapists and doctors had come in over the many weeks Kevin had spent in this teaching hospital. Every shift change, morning and evening, brought different caregivers. My brother's case was interesting, a challenge, and the parade of interns became a blur of murmuring, perplexed voices that rarely addressed him directly. Although the whiteboard on the wall noted that he preferred to be called Kevin, his middle name, those who spoke to him called him by his unused first name, Bruce, then shook their heads at his lack of response.

Then came the afternoon when Andrea blew into his room.

"Hello, Kevin," she sang out. "What can I do for you today?" As she adjusted his tubings and took note of this and that, she leaned over him and listened to his soft reply.

"I'd just feel so much better if I could have a shower," he said.

"I don't see why you can't. A good shampoo would perk you up, I expect."

I looked at my sister and we grinned. Kevin had been asking for a shower for weeks. Everyone said he was too weak, that it would be unmanageable. They had occasionally squirted some gel on his head, covered it with a plastic cap and massaged it in. One aide had rubbed his head so hard he hadn't asked since.

"Before your shower, would you like to take a ride?"

Andrea stepped out and returned minutes later with an empty wheelchair and another patient riding in one beside her. We watched in awe as she expertly assisted our brother from his bed to the chair. Her fingers snapped tubes apart and repositioned them around an IV pole attached to the chair. She hung a couple of monitors over the back and threw a blanket around Kevin's lap and shoulders.

Andrea motioned for my sister Linda to push Kevin. She grabbed the other patient's handlebars, and the five of us strolled the long hall of the ICU, heads down, furtively passing the glass walls of patient rooms and trotting past the nurse's station.

We heard somebody call, "Where are you going with him?" but Andrea just waved and said, "Out for air. We'll be back in twenty minutes!" She never slowed her stride. Linda and I stole a sideways glance at each other and smiled. I felt like we were making a jailbreak and we half expected a siren to sound and a flurry of security guards to chase us. Andrea pushed the elevator button and we were soon in the lobby.

Kevin said not a word. But he lifted his head as we exited the building, his eyes open wide.

Our little troupe halted in the hospital courtyard where my sister and I had often taken our lunches, short breaks from the confines of the room where all the whirring machines took over. Andrea wheeled her charges, along with my sister and me, into a loose circle that reminded me of the wagon trains of the Old West, united against harm. My heart pounded and I wondered how my brother's heart was taking it all. His monitor blinked steadily.

As the nurse, the other patient, and my sister conversed, I watched Kevin. His head tilted back and his gaze turned toward the sky. A look of amazement shone over his whole face. He watched fluffy white clouds drift lazily, with all the time in the world. I knew then he'd thought he would never see the sky again, never be outside that stifling room.

Linda told stories about Kevin's life — how despite his frail health he worked three jobs while they raised their two sons. How his wit and humor were legendary. How he was involved in his community, in his church. How he loved and was loved.

Andrea spoke about how she liked to think of her patients' lives before their illnesses brought them to her. Her duties, she said, included helping them feel better in spirit and body, recognizing them as individuals who needed needles and hospital trappings, but who also needed to be themselves in spite of having to compromise activity and self-sufficiency.

After twenty minutes, she announced the time and patted the hands of both men. Kevin asked softly, "A little longer, please?"

Ten minutes later we paraded back up the elevator.

Heads at the nurse's station snapped our way, as all five of us held our heads high with new vigor. Andrea parked Kevin inside his door as she delivered the other man to his room. We heard the charge nurse call out to her, and it was a few minutes before she returned with two aides who put Kevin in bed. Andrea re-attached all the wires and reset all the machines.

When Andrea finally stood and smoothed her uniform, he reached for her hand. "That was quite a trip," he smiled.

"I'll be back after you've rested a bit, and we'll get that shower."

We three siblings sat in stunned reverence. Then Linda and I described how the sparrows and finches, used to being fed crumbs by visitors and staff, often joined us when we had our courtyard lunches. Kevin could picture it all now that he had been there.

When Andrea returned, I asked her how she would manage to get our brother into the shower and wash his hair. "I'll just get wet too!" was her happy reply. Linda and I went to dinner and when we came back Kevin was clean, refreshed and smiling.

The next day I bought chocolates for Andrea before heading in to visit. She wasn't there. I asked the desk clerk how I could get them to her and was told no one knew where she'd been assigned that day.

She didn't return to the ICU again while we were there.

We asked other caregivers to take Kevin out. "Oh no," they said, "not with all the care he requires; it would be too much for him." We asked for him to be showered. The responses were the same. Most days, for the next week or so, he was allowed to sit in a chair in his room for a few minutes at a time. Three staff members picked him up and moved gingerly with much trepidation and effort. I tried to position his chair to face the window, but it was explained to me that his tubes and wires wouldn't reach that far.

Andrea had fulfilled our hope. She put the sparkle back into my brother's eyes. She assessed the needs of the man as well as the patient and met them. We had her for only one day, but on that day she exceeded her professional mission and became our own personal angel of mercy.

~Marcia Gaye

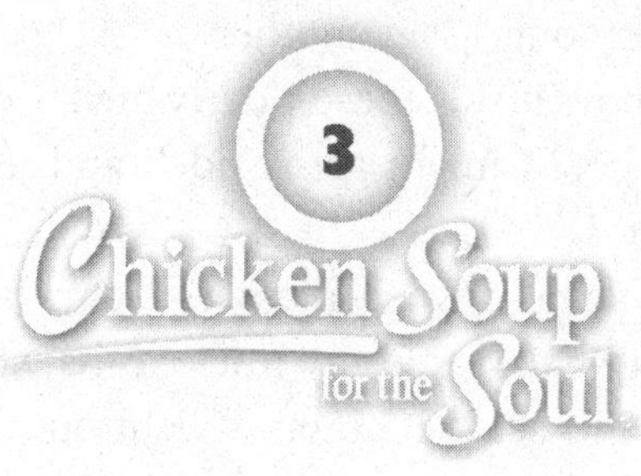

Confession of a Nurse

Today was good. Today was fun. Tomorrow is another one.
~Dr. Seuss

A heavy snowfall covered the ground of the nursing home as I pulled into the parking lot. On Saturday mornings the facility was quieter, without all the office personnel and sales representatives. I enjoyed weekends and looked forward to working as the charge nurse on the men's wing. My Big Boys, as I called them, were always trying to pull pranks on me.

The Big Boys sat in the men's lounge with the television blaring. I loved the stories these retired farmers and men of various occupations told. There were doctors and businessmen alike enjoying the questions I asked them about their youths. My question this day was, "Did you like to play in the snow when you were young?"

All of them had a story to tell about the snowmen they built or the games they played in the snow. They told stories about building forts and having snowball fights. They told stories of their cars stuck in the snow and demonstrated the depth of the snow with their aging hands.

"I haven't felt snow in many years," said Stanley from his wheelchair. The men gazed longingly out the large picture window. One of them remarked. "With the sun on the snow like that, it makes good snow packing."

"Snow won't last long," said another.

I saw the little boys inside these elderly men. I wondered… could I… dared I? Why not? I might get scolded and reprimanded, but I would not get fired.

I gathered up some huge containers from the kitchen and an empty clean garbage can. I told my nurse techs what I was about to do and asked them to get me a mop. I went out the back door and filled all the containers with snow. I took the first container of snow inside to Stanley. "Do you remember making a snowball?"

Stanley smiled, reached, took a handful of the snow and began forming a ball.

"Who would you like to throw it at?" I asked.

"Tom!" Stanley shouted as he tossed the ball at the man near the door. Then all the men got into the action. Workers passed snow to everyone and we all became victims.

"Better duck!" one man warned.

Catch this one!" another challenged.

Raucous laughter echoed throughout the men's wing.

The fights lasted until the snow was melted and the tile floor looked like a water line had broken. The slightly damp men sat grinning as we mopped up the water and handed out towels and warm blankets. Their smiles and energy radiated throughout the day.

I knew when some of them told their families they had thrown snowballs and played with snow, the relatives would laugh and think, "He's confused today."

No, on the contrary, he's alive and witty and well.

~Beverly LaHote Schwind

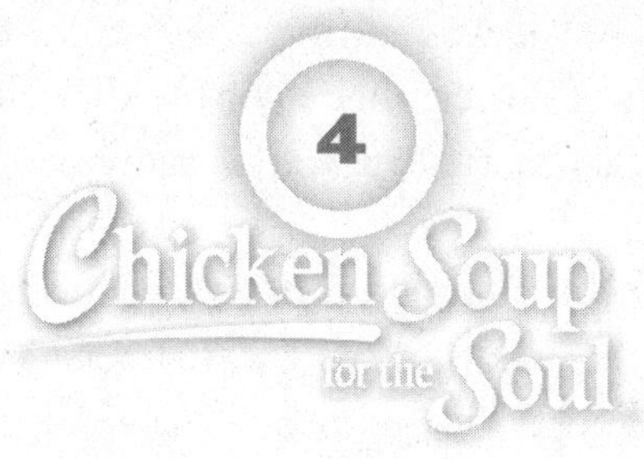

"What Does Your Mom Do?"

The roots of all goodness lie in the soil of appreciation for goodness.
~Dalai Lama

When you're a kid, you come to expect a basic series of questions every time you are introduced to a non-relative. Most were easy: "How old are you?" "What grade are you in?" "What do you want to be when you grow up?" But there was one question that stumped me: "What do your parents do?" Clueless as to the specifics of my parents' jobs, I did my best to fake it.

Dad was a computer programmer, so that one was easy enough. "My dad works on computers," I would say. But mom's job was trickier to explain. She called herself a "nurse practitioner," a term that rolled around in my mouth like marbles. Mom simplified it for me. "Just tell them I teach nursing," she said. "My mom teaches nurses," I would parrot.

When that led to even more questions, I shortened my response to, "My mom's a nurse," though I was ultimately left wondering what it was she actually did. It definitely demanded a lot of time and energy and, between her office at a community college and her long days of "clinicals" (whatever that meant), it seemed her work was important to a lot of people. But it was during a late-night trip with Mom to a hospital in Central Phoenix that I got my first clue as to what she actually did, and what that meant to the many people she referred to as her "patience."

Mom was called in to make rounds unexpectedly that night. It was dark out, near my bedtime, so I was shocked when she asked if I wanted to come along.

I loved the way the light from the streetlamps passed through the car as if on a track whenever I had the privilege of riding after sundown. Anxious to please and in awe of the view from the front seat, I didn't say much. The radio was on low, tuned to some soft rock station, and I didn't touch the dial.

Mom was tense as she guided me through the parking garage and led me to a small emergency waiting room. There were no windows—only a row of white and teal chairs along each wall, a single gray circular end table made of cheap coated plywood, and a mounted TV, the kind that was three feet deep and weighed roughly three hundred pounds.

My mom, her jaw clenched, handed me a bag of peanut M&M's and told me to be good before disappearing to tend to her students and those they cared for in the emergency wing of the hospital. I was a naturally loquacious child and, since this was before ADD diagnosis was common, I was simply deemed "easily bored" by most adults.

My feet swung about a half-inch above the floor as I sat eating candies in the over-lit waiting room. It was cold so I tucked my arms into my shirt and pulled my knees to my chest to keep warm. I studied the only other person in the waiting room, a young black man, out of the corner of my eye, doing my best to make it look like I was watching the news, though the volume was nearly off and I was obviously more of the Nickelodeon cartoons-type.

He wore a dark T-shirt, jeans, and pristine red and white sneakers. Though he had just a sprinkling of facial hair, he looked like a grown man, someone who could teach me a thing or two about the world I lived in, or at least the world I lived adjacent to. In retrospect, the guy couldn't have been a day over twenty-one—a kid, really—but to a grade school white boy from the suburbs who thought of MTV as a sort of cool older sibling, this lone black fellow in that Central Phoenix hospital was a hip-hop enigma. Naturally, I engaged him.

"Hi, my name's Craig, what's yours?" I said—my tried and true childhood icebreaker. He told me his name.

"Why are you at the hospital, is someone sick?"

"Yeah," he said, his head hanging.

"Who?"

"My buddy."

"What happened?"

There was some hesitation this time. My new friend rubbed his hands together and tapped his heels against the white tile floor. "Somebody shot him." As he spoke he rubbed the back of his head with one hand. I nearly bit off my own tongue I was so surprised. I had been pretty sure that getting shot only happened to people on TV or in the movies.

"I'm really sorry," I said. "I hope he's okay."

"Me too. Thanks."

I nodded. There was a moment of silence before I changed the subject. It turned out we liked a lot of the same music, which seemed to tickle him a little. He smiled at me for the first time. He mentioned he was hungry, that he had been waiting for a long time, and I tried to share my candy with him, but he declined.

Now, two decades later, I can't remember how it all played out, but I seem to recall my mother trying to give him a five-dollar bill after I introduced them. I think he politely refused, but I know he reached out to shake my hand before I left that night, and he made me feel pretty cool.

On the drive home I asked my mom if she had seen a man who had been shot. She was vague in her response. Then I thought about that young man, possibly dying from a gunshot wound. I said a silent prayer for him and for our mutual friend in the waiting room, and I felt a burst of pride when I realized that when—if—he ever did wake up, my mom would be there. And if not her, then one of her students. He would be okay, I thought; with a little luck, he would be fine.

Then, in a flash, I realized that I was the lucky one. My mom was a real-life superhero in scrubs. She was a nurse practitioner—an educator and a caretaker. A healer. She was a nurse, and what she did made a difference that even a kid could see.

~Craig S. Baker

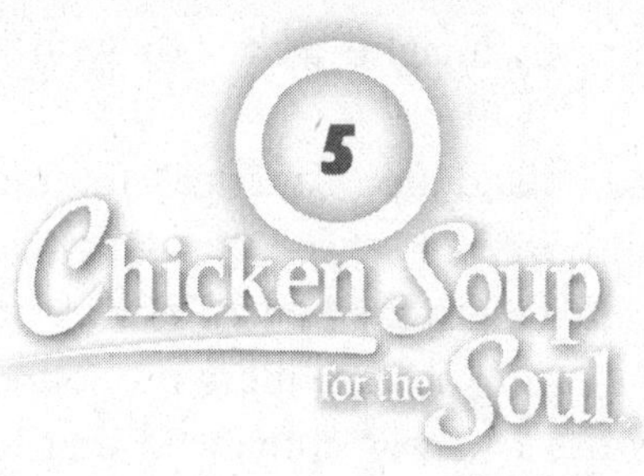

I've Always Been Fond of Nurses

Blessed be the hand that prepares a pleasure for a child, for there is no saying when and where it may bloom forth.
~Douglas Jerrold

My love of nurses began back in 1960. My mother and I were set to board a U.S.-bound military transport ship in Yokosuka, Japan, when a review of our records showed we lacked the proper documentation that would allow us passage. We were traveling without my mother's husband (my newly adoptive father whom I had yet to meet) because he was a navy man and had already been transferred back to the States. Given my mom's limited English and the bureaucratic confluence of customs, immigration, and military regulations, our situation would not find quick relief. When my mom began wiping away tears, I was bewildered, clueless as to what was happening.

I was eager to board the ship and get the journey underway, and spent much of my time in the terminal daydreaming. Like so many young Japanese boys, my heroes either swung samurai swords or baseball bats. I knew that America was where baseball came from, but I also wondered if I would ever see another samurai movie. I had watched my very first John Wayne western, *Rio Bravo*, just months before and realized that the western was very similar to a samurai movie, and I could easily imagine a cowboy with a six-shooter *and* a samurai sword.

My mother had talked up "America" for months, but as she pleaded with the authorities I sensed that America was not too keen on us. When she returned to the bench in the middle of the embarkation terminal, her crying became more pronounced and my bewilderment turned to dread. I was convinced that her sobbing meant we would not only miss the ship, but likely not ever be allowed into America. Clutching my mother's arm, I too began to bawl.

It was at that very moment… as if she were the star making her entrance onto the stage… that a woman walked into the terminal in full nurse uniform and immediately captured everyone's attention. She chatted briefly with a naval officer who directed her our way. As she approached, I tried to hide behind the bench but stumbled and scraped my knee. I peered up over the bench and made eye contact with her just as she scrunched her brow, cocked her head to one side and exaggerated a sad face, then offered up a huge grin. I was enchanted; it was the very first time I ever saw such a woman, a Gaijin with golden blond hair and gem-like blue eyes.

Standing in front of us, she wore a very kind face with soft features that offset her crisply starched uniform. With her white blouse and skirt, she wore white stockings, white shoes, and her golden hair up in a bun that was partially hidden by one of those odd white caps that American nurses don't wear anymore. She was the very model of the registered nurse. When she sat down beside us and began speaking to my mother in Japanese, I saw her as an angel, a beautiful and blithe spirit who, with an arm around Mom's shoulders, comforted her with a warmth and reassurance that proved a gentle salve to my mother's fractured emotions.

Within a few minutes the nurse had Mom smiling as she explained to us that our health records were incomplete, that the officials had to make sure we were not carrying any exotic diseases. The nurse escorted us to the medical dispensary for new physicals. She also put antiseptic on my scraped knee and introduced me to the Band-Aid. Within a couple of hours, we were cleared to board the ship.

I departed for the States that day with three ideas embossed prominently in my brain: 1) baseball is best in America; 2) don't mess with John Wayne without a samurai sword; and 3) if you get hurt playing baseball or messing with John Wayne, find a nurse.

My wife became an RN in her own right a few years after we were married, and whenever I recounted this story, my brunette wife would add jokingly that it also explained why I was so attracted to blondes! But I've always been fond of nurses, all kinds! My wife was too modest to admit that she had helped heal countless physical and emotional wounds throughout her years as a nurse. I have come across many notes, cards, and letters addressed to her from grateful patients and family members deeply touched by her caring.

~Kosuke Vasquez

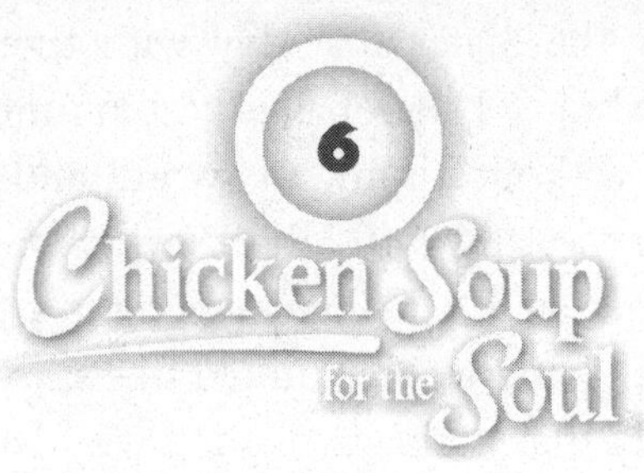

Lip Service

Dear children, let us not love with words or speech, but with actions and in truth.
~1 John 3:18

She walked into the exam room holding her mother's hand tightly. Compared to the dozens of other children we had triaged that sweltering tropical morning at the South American mission hospital, she was quite overdressed. Instead of the expected T-shirt and shorts, she wore a frilly pink dress. Instead of flip-flops, she wore Mary Janes on that wet cement floor that reeked of bleach. A shock of springy curls bounced off her shoulders when she plopped down on a chair before us. Even though she covered her mouth with a rag, the sparkle in her mischievous brown eyes told of a hidden smile.

"Well, hello! What is your name?" Dr. G asked.

I translated the question.

In a voice muffled by the fabric she said, "Maria." Her nasal twang was distinctive of an uncorrected cleft defect.

Dr. G asked, "May I examine you, Maria?" He pulled a penlight from his lab coat pocket. I handed him a tongue depressor.

Maria shuffled around on her chair. "My mom says if you fix me I can go to school." With the rag still firmly pressed over her mouth she asked, "It's true?"

The mother searched our faces, her eyes filled with hope. We could hear the desperation in her voice when she asked, "Can you help my girl?" With trembling hands she smoothed Maria's hair. "All she wants is to go to school… to play like other children." Lowering her voice she continued, "Children are afraid of her. Some call her very bad names."

A fan hummed next to an open window, pushing the humid air around. Fragments of conversations, children's laughter, and infant's cries drifted inside the room. Outside, parents waited in line for hours hoping their children would be selected for surgery.

"Well, let's have the doctor take a look then, okay?" Gently I moved the rag away from the girl's face. The severe cleft defect split from her upper lip through the base of her nose. Since birth the child had never had treatments. However we had seen many other patients with even worse defects. Some had deformities that included the gum line, whether unilateral or bilateral, and their teeth grew in grotesque angles from protruding gums. Others had palate defects only, and many had a combination of unilateral or bilateral fissures including cleft palates.

Dr. G shone the light into the gaping hole in the girl's face. "Palate's intact. Fissure's on the right."

I noted Dr. G's assessments on the surgery scheduling form.

Dr. G clicked off the penlight, winked at Maria and said, "We'll see you in a couple of days then, young lady."

Before I had a chance to finish translating Dr. G's sentence, the mother embraced me, crying out, "Thank you, thank you!"

Clapping with excitement, Maria laughed. This made the gap between her upper-lip widen and lobes of pink tissue dangled at each side of her mouth. Instantly she covered it with the rag.

We continued to see patients throughout the day, from infants and toddlers to school aged children, to teenagers and young adults, and even a fifty-six-year-old woman. There were multiple types and severity levels of maxillofacial deformities. And it was with careful consideration that Dr. G, the anesthesia provider, and the local medical team made the difficult decisions about which patients would be selected for surgery and which would be turned away.

Thirty-one patients were selected and scheduled for surgery.

Maria and her mother arrived almost an hour early on the day of her operation. It was my teenage daughter's first mission trip. Since her job was to distribute toys and play with the children, she and Maria soon became friends, coloring pictures and playing with the other children in the pre-operative area.

When the time came to wheel Maria's stretcher toward the OR, she waved a groggy goodbye to her inconsolable mother, all the while keeping the rag over her lips.

We lifted the child onto the OR table. The anesthetist gently removed the rag from her face and placed the oxygen mask over her mouth and nose. Her long eyelashes fluttered as medication was administered through her IV. Her skin was prepped, and sterile green towels were placed around her head and face. Disposable drapes covered her tiny frame. Dr. G adjusted the overhead lights and began the operation, then finally connected both sides of the lip like two perfectly aligned puzzle pieces.

When Maria was wheeled into the recovery room, her mother rushed to meet us. With both hands covering her face she sobbed. "My girl, Maria. You are beautiful!"

Maria was still sedated, but awake enough when I placed a handheld mirror before her face. "Look, Maria. What do you think?"

With glassy eyes she took the mirror from my hand. For several seconds she stared at her image. Suddenly, with a gasp, she said, "I can go to school now."

Many days later, on the last day of the mission trip, exhausted but elated, we packed our equipment and supplies. All we wanted was some food, a shower, and rest before our eight-hour-plus flight home the following day. But instead we were invited by one of the nurses to visit her church service. We politely attempted to beg off, but she refused to accept any of our excuses. Sweaty and hungry, we reluctantly put on our lab coats over our scrubs, and followed her to a waiting van.

The church was packed when we arrived, but there was a reserved pew in front for the medical team. To our surprise the service had been planned by the community to thank us.

The pastor prayed over our team, and then came the altar call. We bowed our heads to a familiar hymn sung in the congregation's native tongue. A large crowd gathered at the altar. Suddenly from within the group, a blur of pink satin and bouncing curls rushed toward us. I pulled at Dr. G's sleeve, and he opened his eyes. Maria stood before him with arms wide open, her perfect smile marred only by a blue suture line. Overcome with emotion, Dr. G swooped up the child in his arms. This moment brought the entire trip into perspective for all of us.

Our mission was to bless the underprivileged with surgery, or so we thought.

But in reality God blessed us through the humbleness and faithfulness of that poor, but joyous, community.

Everything else was just lip service.

~Ivani Martucci Greppi

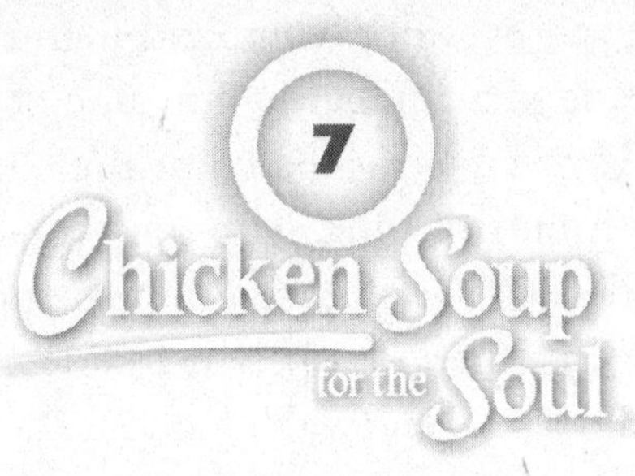

I Understand

Our prime purpose in this life is to help others.
~Dalai Lama

"Are you crazy? You finally retired! Why would you want to work in a hospital again?" My friends couldn't understand why, after forty years of nursing and four of retirement, I would return to nursing. Actually, I didn't understand either. Tired of the daily commute and pressures of the job, I had eagerly and joyfully retired with no plans to practice nursing again.

Then one day a friend who was also a retired nurse told me how much she loved being a part of the Volunteer Registered Nurse program. "You help nurses care for patients at the bedside," she said, "and the best part is, you do so at your own speed."

She directed me to the program at our local hospital, and after completing lots of paperwork and a few classes, I was excited about getting back to the bedside. On my first day, after a short orientation, I stepped onto the surgical floor to be welcomed with smiles and hellos from the staff. I checked with the charge nurse to see who needed my help the most or if there was a particular patient requiring some extra care. The charge nurse directed me to a patient care tech who was obviously overwhelmed.

She smiled. "I am so glad to see you. I can't believe you are here to help me." Taking a deep breath, she added, "Mr. Jones needs a bath and some extra attention. He is so disappointed he's not going home today."

I proceeded to the patient's room to see a sad man staring out the window.

I gave him my biggest smile. "Hi, I'm Mary, a volunteer RN and I'm here to take special care of you this morning."

I asked if he would like to take a shower and he shook his head glumly.

"Taking a shower and putting on clean pajamas may make you feel better," I encouraged.

He agreed and walked to the shower while I made his bed with fresh linen and tidied his room. When he finished his shower, I said, "How would you like a foot-soak while you sit in your chair?"

"That would be wonderful," he said.

As he soaked his feet we had a chance to talk about his diagnosis and his disappointment at not being able to go home. I expressed my sympathy and explained the possible reason he needed to stay a day longer. I helped dry his feet and massaged them with lotion.

"Is there anything else I can do for you?"

"No, I believe you have done a great deal. Thank you. I feel so much better than when you came in here. I can't thank you enough."

My heart leaped. I felt I had made a small difference. But I was not done yet.

I found the patient care tech with another patient who had just returned from the OR. As I entered I saw a small frail man. His voice was weak but his eyes were bright. I took his vital signs, as directed, and documented them on a "sticky note." The PCT was encouraging him to eat something from the lunch tray in front of him. It was obvious he had no strength in his arms or crippled hands to raise a Styrofoam cup or use a spoon.

"You're busy with other patients," I told her. "I'll help him."

"Are you sure?"

"Of course. That is what I am here for."

I fed him a Popsicle in a Styrofoam cup, then offered him broth and Jell-O.

"Yuck!" he said.

So I got him some hot tea with two packs of sweetener and held the cup to his lips as he sipped. It was too hot at first, so between sips we talked about the facility where he lived and his doctor's promise that he would go back there after this simple procedure.

He finished his tea and said, "There are too many blankets on me; they're too heavy."

I removed the bedspread and several blankets.

"Uncover my feet," he requested.

So I uncovered his feet.

I frowned when I found two crippled, scaly, shriveled feet.

"Would you like some lotion on your feet?"

"That would feel so good."

I rubbed his feet very gently with soothing cream and covered them with bed socks. Then I covered him with a light warmed blanket and a sheet.

"Can I do anything else for you?"

"How can I reach you? You understand me and a lot of the others don't." My heart burst.

Volunteer nursing is the best "job" I've ever had. I am still a nurse. Now I understand.

~Mary Clary

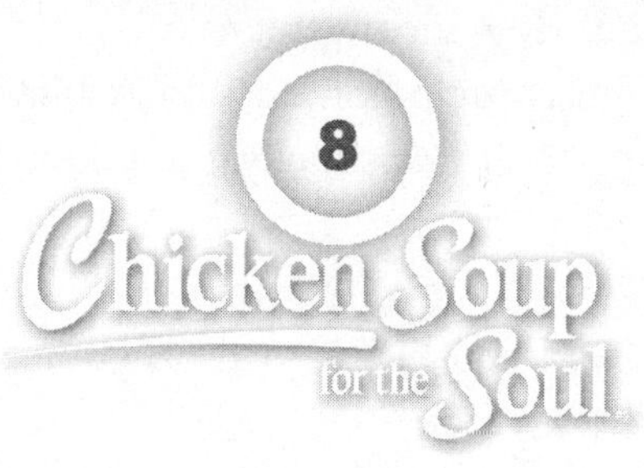

Keeping the Pace

Your greatest danger is letting the urgent things crowd out the important.
~Charles E. Hummel, Tyranny of the Urgent

It was going to be another busy morning. I organized my day and reviewed charts, keeping one eye on the clock's minute hand. Then I headed for the floor. Sigh—blood sugar to check. Another sigh—contact isolation. Pulling on my gown and gloves, I wondered how I could speed up the assessment process. What shortcuts could I take? With today's workload, I needed to pick up the pace.

"Good morning. My name is Glenna. I'll be your nurse. How are you?"

Sally stared at me, expressionless. I remembered that she also had a mental health diagnosis and had been some trouble for the night shift.

Hoping Sally would not disrupt my schedule, I pressed on, listening to her heart and lungs, and checking her skin. As she mumbled I made appropriate "Hmms," and "Ahhs" as though I were really listening to her.

"You don't look very comfortable," I commented. I hoped she didn't want something for pain. Maybe I could get by with repositioning her, saving a trip back to the med room.

"My neck hurts."

I groaned inside. How inconvenient.

"Here, let me get your pillow," I said, while I fluffed and rearranged it. "How's that?" If I was lucky, the pillow trick would satisfy her.

"It still hurts."

I relented. "Would you like me to rub your neck?" I sighed as I looked at the merciless clock.

She nodded. I quietly started to massage her neck, thinking about how much time this would cost me.

My thoughts jolted to a stop when she said, "Isn't that what nurses do?"

My brain went ballistic. *Are you kidding? Who has time for neck rubs? Doesn't she realize I have four other patients waiting for me? I can't afford the time for a neck rub!* I thought about assessments, charting, med passes, audits, documentation, JCAHO… I caught my breath and half-smiled. Sally was right.

I relaxed and gently, lovingly rubbed the tense muscles of her neck. "Yes, this is what nurses do." I gulped. "Sally, would you like a warm blanket?"

~Glenna J. Eady

This story first appeared in *Our Stories: Living the Adventist Health Message Volume II*. We want to thank Adventist Health for allowing us to share it.

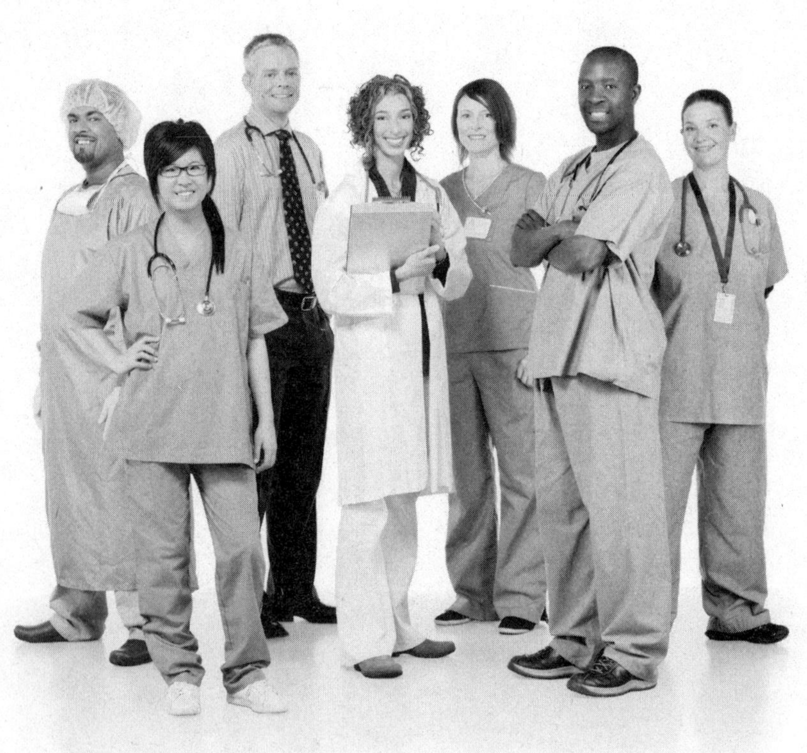

Inspiration for Nurses

Defining Moments

When you are inspired by some great purpose, some extraordinary project, all of your thoughts break their bonds, your mind transcends limitations, your consciousness expands in every direction, and you find yourself in a new, great and wonderful world. Dormant forces, faculties and talents become alive and you discover yourself to be a greater person than you ever dreamed yourself to be.

~Indian Philosopher Patanjali

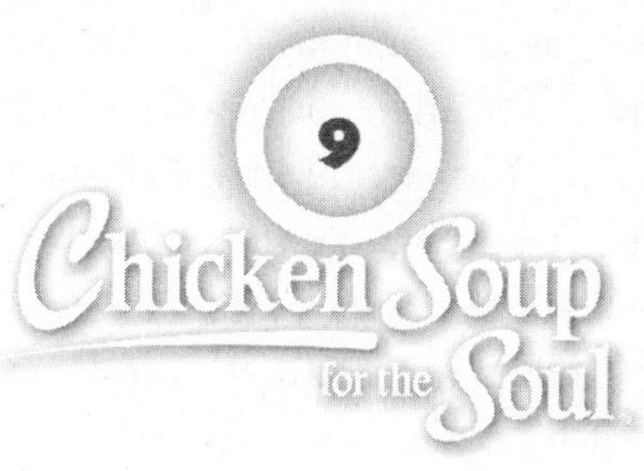

Change of Heart

Beautiful young people are accidents of nature, but beautiful old people are works of art.
~Eleanor Roosevelt

It broke my heart to leave the Post-Anesthesia Care Unit (PACU) where I'd been happily employed for fifteen years. The staff was great, all good friends who worked well together. We were a unit of proud critical care nurses with tremendous responsibility. Our green scrubs and the stethoscopes dangling from our necks marked us as "important people." But then my job, with all its glory and challenges, came to a screeching halt when my husband accepted employment out of state.

Changing jobs is never easy but I felt certain I'd find another PACU that wanted someone with my credentials. Two weeks of job searching and interviewing proved me dead wrong. I found no openings for post-anesthesia care nurses. How could this be? I was devastated.

After one more disappointing rejection the nurse recruiter politely suggested I try the hospital's CCC unit across the street. I had no idea what CCC stood for until I saw the sign: Continuing Care Center. I stared at the sign and cringed. Obviously CCC was an elaborate name for a nursing home! Working in a nursing home certainly did not fit into my career plans.

My view of nursing homes had been defined by a one-time visit with a youth group as a teenager. I vividly recalled dreary halls, dreadful odors, and unfortunate old people curled in a fetal position waiting for life to end. My mental image of the nursing staff wasn't much better. I perceived the nurses to be rather dull, not too spiffy or sharp. Not top quality like me.

Since I already had an appointment I followed through and met with the director of nurses at the CCC. She quickly skimmed my references and indicated I might fit into their float pool. How strange. She made it sound like a privilege to work there.

A tour revealed a clean, odor-free building. In fact, the place was brightly decorated and attractive. I took the job, planning to keep an eye on the want ads for something better suited to my skills.

Orientation proved to be another eye opener. The instructor was an ex-Navy nurse who stressed excellence. She had no tolerance for sloppy work or idleness. A six-page test to evaluate my skills not only intimidated me but caused me to wonder if I'd pass. My mental image of a low-caliber staff rapidly changed.

Once on the unit, more evidence blew holes in my preconceived notions. Three staffers had been ICU nurses and two had been PACU nurses. Imagine that! I also learned that several of the RNs were new graduates specializing in geriatrics. The nurses were top-notch all the way. They proved to me that critical care nurses didn't hold a monopoly on quality care. I secretly hoped I could measure up to their standards.

I swallowed my now battered pride and depended on the nurses to teach me the unit's routine. My snobby attitude toward nursing home personnel changed. With their friendly manner and efficient skills they helped ease me into the daily assignments.

Another surprise awaited me when I met the residents. Most of the patients in the PACU were groggy from anesthesia so I seldom had verbal interaction. I found the elderly residents in the CCC to be delightful as they shared their life stories and told corny jokes. Most of all I admired their strength and unlimited courage in the face of hardship. Since many of them were admitted for the long haul, I was also able to develop a close relationship with them and their families.

I had worked there only a few weeks when one of my favorite residents needed to be discharged. When her family came to take her home, she pulled me close and said with her Polish accent, "You have been good to me. I will miss you." I struggled to hold back my tears.

At that moment I knew I was hooked. The residents and staff had become part of me. I no longer checked the want ads in the newspaper for another job because the nursing home, by whatever name, was where I belonged… my career plans fulfilled.

~Barbara Brady

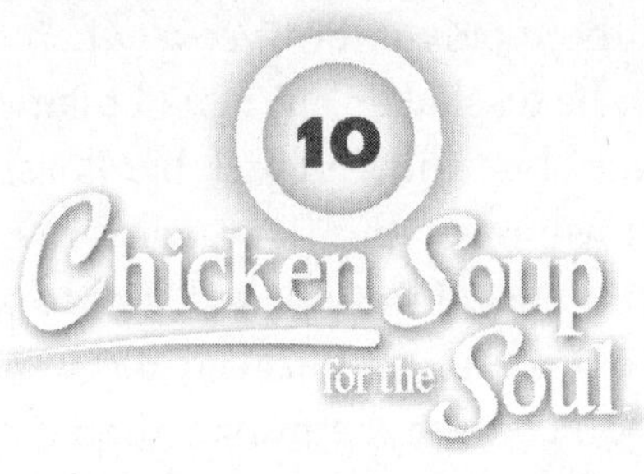

Graduation Day

Love one another and help others to rise to the higher levels, simply by pouring out love. Love is infectious and the greatest healing energy.
~Sai Baba

"One teenage girl is dead and another is in critical condition following a Sunday night shooting in Cambridge." This was the lead in *The Cambridge Chronicle* on June 4, 2012. Both victims were students at Cambridge Rindge and Latin School where I am a school nurse. In this inconceivable tragedy, Shay lost her life. Thanialee, the survivor, was shot several times and hospitalized at Mass General in Boston.

Graduation was in three days, and as I headed to the hospital to visit her, I recalled how excited Thanialee had been two weeks earlier when I chaperoned prom. She'd literally beamed about being a senior and counted the days until graduation, then danced all night long.

Through the IVs, machines, and tubes, I took her hand. Her mother held her other hand as Thanialee said hoarsely, "I miss school, my friends." Tears filled her eyes. "And I'll miss graduation."

"It's okay to cry," I whispered. I gave her all of the emotional support I had and I left feeling angry, sad, and useless.

Then, one of my colleagues had an idea. What if Thanialee could attend her graduation via Skype? What if I could do something positive that could change her outlook on her life, if even for a few hours?

Determined, I met with the IT specialists at the hospital and the school. They explained how we could make this happen. I volunteered to get the equipment, and that very afternoon I borrowed a $30,000 five-foot-tall robot and carefully loaded it into my SUV. I made my way back to the high school, where the hospital IT specialist joined me. We positioned the robot/computer on stage in the dignitary section and dressed it in a cap and gown. While the technical aspects were being worked out for the robot to help project Thanialee live on the big screen, I was in the upstairs gym working with our IT specialist getting my iPad to synch with the robot/computer in her hospital room. If this worked, she would be able to participate in the pre-graduation flower pinning reception too.

It was touch and go for a while as we worked feverishly to get the connections and audio to work. Then, like magic, we saw Thanialee in her hospital bed! We tested it several times to make sure it would not fail, and at 4:30 p.m. the school IT specialist had to leave and I was on my own. Nervously, I watched the clock tick to 5:00. I launched the Skype session and Thanialee appeared on my screen, smiling through tears, dressed in her cap and gown.

We shared a few heartfelt words, and then it was time for the students to talk with their classmate. Thanialee spent an hour with her classmates. "I love you!" they chimed repeatedly, back and forth. I could hardly hold back my own tears of joy during this love fest. The students were ecstatic about having Thanialee participate in this upbeat, beautiful celebration.

By then it was 6:00. Graduation time! The big equipment on the stage took over. The ceremony started with a moment of silence for Shay, with sniffles and muffled sobs breaking the hush. There was another moment of silence and hope for Thanialee.

Then, to everyone's surprise, the principal announced, "Thanialee is with us tonight via video conferencing!" At that moment her face appeared on the large screen on the stage. The entire gym vibrated with clapping, cheering and screaming. Thanialee waved and said, "I love you," then began the chant. "Seniors! Seniors!" The gym reverberated with her classmates cheering, "Seniors! Seniors! Seniors!"

It was powerful. Then, as planned, the screen went back to black as the graduation proceeded. Thanialee continued to have the live feed in her hospital room throughout the ceremony.

After all the other graduates had been called, Thanialee's tenth-grade brother marched on stage to accept her diploma. This time the crowd went even wilder. They quieted only to see and hear Thanialee one last time on the screen.

"Congratulations, everyone. I love you all so much. Thank you for our amazing graduation… together." Her mother came on briefly too, offering her thanks for all the love and support.

As the ceremony came to a close, happiness and joy radiated throughout the entire gymnasium. Somehow the heaviness we were all feeling had lifted.

Although this was one of the saddest tragedies in my career, that graduation was one of the highlights of my nursing profession. School nursing is so much more than bandaging bodies: it's mending the minds and soothing the spirits of students and parents, too.

~Tracy Rose-Tynes

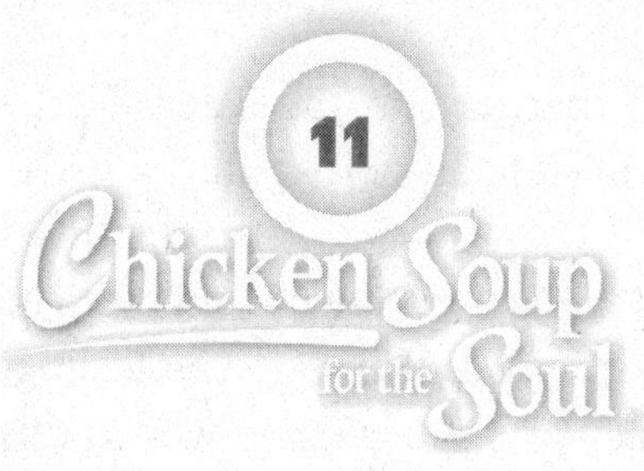

The Bus Stop

Appreciation is a wonderful thing. It makes what is excellent in others belong to us as well.
~Voltaire

Mom and I walked side by side through town. I was twelve years old, dependent on her, yet wanting so much to be my own person. She raised me by herself, her only child, and except for when I was at school we were almost always together.

Before I was born she had worked as a nurse, but she stopped shortly after my birth to care for me. Recently she had returned to work at the local hospital.

I didn't like her going back to work. She left at 5:45 a.m., which left me responsible for waking myself up, fixing breakfast, and walking to the 7:30 a.m. bus.

I hated being left home alone in the mornings, but I especially hated having to take the bus. Once I had missed it, and I wasn't only late to school, but I had caused Mom to scramble to find someone else to drive me. After that I was so worried I would miss the bus that I left way too early every day to make the half-mile walk. I stood by myself before the other kids arrived, in rain, sleet and snow, in agonizing preteen embarrassment as commuters drove by.

Mom worked the day shift so she could pick me up after school. On days she didn't go to the hospital, she drove me both ways. Those were the best days.

As we walked that day on the sidewalk, I saw an older man approaching us. He suddenly broke into a wide smile, but I didn't recognize him.

"Leigh! Leigh!" he said, calling my mother's name.

"Hello," she responded. "How are you feeling?"

"Couldn't be better! Thanks. Now who is this lovely young person?" he asked jovially.

"This is my daughter," Mom replied, looking over to me. "Jenny, can you say hello?"

I looked at him and smiled, unsure of my role.

"Well, it is very nice to meet you, young lady. I hope you know how lucky you are!" he said.

I looked at him uncertainly since I had no idea what he was talking about and I didn't feel lucky at all, especially since he was standing too close to me.

"You have the most wonderful, caring and lovely mother," he said over-enunciating the words. "When I was in the hospital last month she took the best care of me. She made every day better. Every day. In fact, young lady, I shall never forget her."

He removed his attention from me and went back to addressing my mother.

I watched this stranger's delight in my mom. He kept thanking her and thanking her.

Right then it dawned on me what it meant for my mom to be a nurse, what it actually meant for her to go and do her job while I was at school. She was caring for, serving, and loving random strangers, often during some of the scariest times in their lives.

It wasn't the last time I witnessed someone thanking Mom or complimenting her on her bedside manner, but it was the first time I understood why I stood at the bus stop every morning. My mom was a nurse, and sometimes life was about other people. She cared for them… and me, too.

~Jennifer Quasha

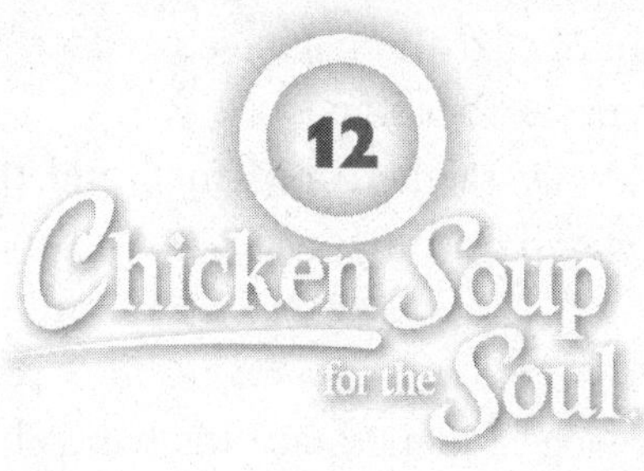

A Measure of Love

Being deeply loved by someone gives you strength; loving someone deeply gives you courage.
~Lao Tzu

“Come with me.” Dr. Warren, a pediatric oncologist, strode toward the patient room I had left just a minute earlier. I squelched a sigh, turned around and followed him in.

I was a newly minted registered nurse and this was my second week in Pediatrics. I’d envisioned myself on an adult medical-surgical floor at this hospital where I’d done my clinical training, but the only vacancy had been in this unit. So I swallowed my fears about working with children and took the job.

The patient, fourteen-year-old Janice, sat propped up on pillows. Her parents watched the doctor. Her mother’s trembling fingers wrapped around her necklace while her father paced between Janice’s bed and the empty one next to the door. He stopped when Dr. Warren entered.

I stood by the door clenching my hands behind my back, ready to dash out of the room at the first opportunity. Besides needing to pass meds, I had five other patients who needed care.

Dr. Warren asked the parents to take a seat. Janice’s mother did so, but her father refused. He demanded, “What’s the verdict, Doctor?”

Dr. Warren opened Janice’s chart. In a low, we’ve-done-all-we-can-do voice, he informed them Janice's cancer was back and had spread. He offered no further hope.

The room suddenly seemed too small and the air too heavy. I fidgeted with my watch and my eyes scanned the bedside table for the box of tissues.

Janice's mother gasped.

Her husband's face reddened and his hands balled into fists. He glared at the doctor. "Get out."

"Daddy!" Janice's raspy voice was barely above a whisper.

Dr. Warren held up his hand, "Mr. Barnes, I can understand how devastating this is, but..."

"No. No, you can't." The dad's voice broke and he stepped toward Janice. Husband and wife stood like sentries on either side of her bed. "Just leave us with our daughter. Please."

Dr. Warren frowned and I thought he'd try to persuade the parents to put their emotions aside momentarily. Instead he checked his watch and said, "I'll give you some time. We'll discuss it later." With that he spun around and slipped past me out the door.

I froze. I'd never dealt with a dying patient. Even in nursing school I'd been the student with those lucky patients who were admitted, treated, and released. In a tiny voice, I asked, "Would you like me to leave too?"

Mr. Barnes ignored me. His wife, tears streaming down her face, sat silently on the edge of Janice's bed, embraced her daughter and rocked back and forth. Fearing I'd start to cry too, I hustled out of the room.

In the hallway, I blew out a breath and the lump in my throat dissolved. I shook off the sorrow I felt for the Barnes family and proceeded to pass the rest of my meds. As I did so, though, the niggling feeling that I hadn't done my best for Janice and her family snuck up on me. I completed my charting, then reluctantly returned to her room.

Her father was nowhere to be seen, but her mother sat on a chair next to the bed, holding Janice's hand in silence. Both looked up.

"Can I do anything for you?" Such an inane question. What could

I do for a dying girl and her mother?

Mrs. Barnes pushed her hair back from her face. "I'm sorry my husband flew off the handle like that."

I was surprised by her apology. I should've been the one apologizing for escaping from the room. "It's understandable." I really was unsure what to say and was uncomfortable with the silence, so I blurted out, "Would you like me to page Dr. Warren now?"

"Not yet." Mrs. Barnes stroked Janice's cheek. "My husband is in the cafeteria. I think I'll join him." She gently asked her daughter, "Will you be all right while I'm there?" Janice nodded and Mrs. Barnes rose and kissed her. "Be back real soon."

That left me alone with my patient. We stumbled through a short, stilted conversation. I desperately hoped her parents would return quickly. Janice, looking out the window, said, "I'm their only kid. My parents are taking this hard."

I said a quick, silent prayer that my reply wouldn't make things worse. "They must love you a lot."

She nodded. "Yeah." She looked at me with dark eyes that contrasted with her pale skin. "I think they're afraid. You know, about what it's gonna be like."

I glanced at my watch and reminded myself I had other patients. But I didn't want to leave Janice just then. "Be like?"

"You know, when I'm gone." She said it so matter-of-factly she could have been talking about her family's long-dead pet. "But I'm not. Scared, I mean."

Just then her parents returned and asked me to page Dr. Warren. After doing so, I went about caring for my other patients.

At the end of my shift, I was still thinking about Janice and was eager to talk to her more.

The next morning in report I heard that her parents wanted everything done for their daughter, despite Dr. Warren's prognosis. My heart grew heavy knowing all that the girl would have to endure, only to succumb to the cancer anyway. I made my way to her room where she lay half-awake.

"Good morning, Janice. Just need to take your temperature."

She struggled to sit up. "My mom and dad want me to have all that awful stuff again."

"How are you with that?"

She shrugged. "I don't want it. I'm gonna die anyway."

"Did you tell them that?"

"Couldn't. It's important to them."

I cocked my head. "You're going to go through that so *they* feel better?"

She nodded. "When I'm dead… " Her voice caught, but she went on. "They didn't say it, but I think they want to feel like, you know…"

"Like they did everything?"

"Yeah. They'll feel better."

I told myself to keep quiet, but I couldn't stop. "What about how you feel?"

She struggled with the next words. "It's okay. I'll be dead soon. They have the rest of their lives to deal with me being gone."

I fought back tears, amazed at the measure of her love for her parents. "You're very brave."

She shrugged, then slid back down into the pillow. "I'm really tired now. I'm going to sleep."

The rest of my day was busy and I only had time to pop in her room, say hello to her parents, and check vitals and her IV. I was off the next day, but when I returned the day after, I learned Janice had passed away, her family by her side. I wondered if, because she was selflessly willing to endure more pain for love of her parents, God hadn't given her the gift of a quick, relatively easy death.

I think back now to Janice and am still humbled by the girl's willingness to sacrifice herself for the sake of love. While her parents had done everything they could for her, she had done everything she could for them.

~Carole Fowkes

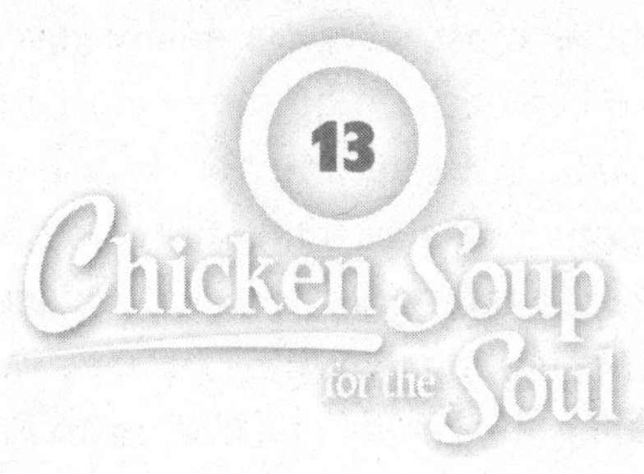

The Maintenance Man

Each person has an ideal, a hope, a dream which represents the soul. We must give to it the warmth of love, the light of understanding and the essence of encouragement.
~Colby Dorr Dam

I was wary of him. He hung around, repeatedly cleaning the kitchen area of the staff room as my students gathered their belongings at the end of their shifts. I worried he was checking out "my girls." His head was usually down, but it seemed he was eavesdropping on their conversations.

As a clinical instructor, I worked with nursing students on a medical floor on the evening shifts. We wrapped up around 9:30 p.m. and then the students convened in a crowded staff room for a bit of their own de-briefing, joking around, exchanging e-mail addresses, or taking group selfies. As they'd pack up their backpacks, notes, and various electronic devices, laughter emanated from the small group.

I suppose it's natural that we instructors watch out for our little flocks when students might be oblivious to who's watching them. There was no reason to expect anything suspicious; the man had appropriate identification, but I tended to be on the cautious side.

The students were unique in that they comprised a group of Internationally Educated Nurses (IENs), all of whom had studied and qualified for nursing in their home countries and had immigrated to Canada with the intent to refresh their skills and practice here. They were a joy to teach, as most were extremely eager to complete this clinical portion, the last of the requirements that would allow them to write the Canadian RN exams and apply for positions.

One of my star students was a tall, outgoing woman from South Africa who had recently immigrated. She'd decided to resuscitate her nursing career after spending a number of years raising her children. Her goal was to polish her skills and return to emergency nursing, which was her specialty in South Africa. Since that was my first career, we had a common bond.

She was a white woman with an unusual streak of vibrantly dyed red hair in her otherwise ordinary head of sandy brown. Joyfully, she sung out her friendly greeting of, "Good morning, M'lady," at the beginning of every shift in her lilting Afrikaans accent. She soaked up everything I could possibly offer. She helped the other students on the computers at the hospital and shared her clinical experiences. She got the most out of her clinical rotation because she gave as much or more than anyone else.

Our end-of-shift ritual continued and the dark-skinned maintenance man still hung about. I noted his sad gaze and felt a sense of loss coming from him.

Finally, one evening he approached me after the students had departed. In heavily accented English, he asked, "What program these students in?"

I told him, but wondered where he was going with this. He related how he and his wife had immigrated to Canada just a few years earlier. They had both been RNs in Africa. For eighteen years he was in charge of HIV/AIDS education programs throughout Kenya and other parts of Africa. He had hoped to practice nursing in Canada, but language was a barrier. He was taking English classes. He had heard a bit about the IEN program and was thinking of applying, but admitted his work and study schedule was already taxing. Once he qualified, if he did, his wife was going to try to regain her RN qualifications too.

I smiled at my own misconceptions about this experienced African nurse who had obviously made a huge impact in his homeland. Ever the ambassador for the college, I told him more about the IEN program and how to apply. I encouraged him to continue with his studies and I wished him the best in resuming his nursing career.

After that conversation, he seemed to relax a little more when the students were finishing their shifts, his eyes occasionally lighting up, although often wistful.

My group continued to expand their skills and share many successes. You could feel the excitement in the air as they neared completion of the clinical rotations and anticipated writing their exams.

On one shift in the final week I came in early to find my South African student deep in conversation with the maintenance man in a side conference room, her clear and encouraging voice melding with his quiet responses, his head eventually nodding in comprehension. He looked up to acknowledge me with a shy smile.

"I accepted into the IEN program," he said with a smile. He held his head higher, his eyes lit up, and he carried himself tall with obvious pride.

He had sought out a fellow African upon realizing the first course was on medication. She was conducting a mini-teaching session on IV therapy calculations.

My heart swelled with pride to see the South African woman sharing her knowledge with the Kenyan maintenance man, proving that the language of nursing transcends race, colour, creed, and gender.

~Colleen Stewart Haynes

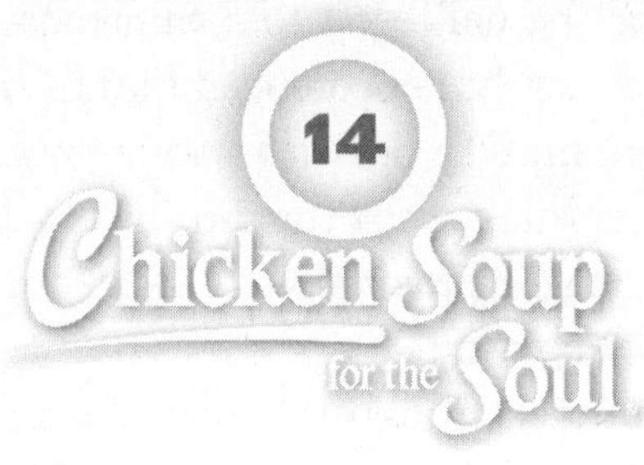

Nocturnal Poet

If you want others to be happy, practice compassion. If you want to be happy, practice compassion.
~*Dalai Lama*

Over forty years ago, as a newly minted RN, I spread my wings to Los Angeles, California. I had been promised a position working days in the ER, my dream job. But when I got there, all that was available was night shift on the orthopedic ward. I took it unhappily, because going home wasn't an option.

I hated night shift and disliked orthopedics. The combination was not a good one for me. I was cranky and I knew it. I tried to make up for it, with only dubious degrees of success.

The ward on which I worked was a curious combination of specialties, orthopedics and isolation. It was a very busy ward and we were understaffed for the patient load. We were constantly running, always behind on just about everything. It was a very stressful way to nurse and we staggered home at the end of every shift thinking that the patients deserved better.

All of which did nothing to reduce my grumpiness.

We gave a lot of medication on nights: lots of painkillers but mainly IV antibiotics. It was hard to give meds quietly in a dark room. I usually woke at least one patient. I'd bump into something, or shine the flashlight too close to someone's eyes. But I tiptoed in and tried as hard as I could to get the antibiotics set up quietly. It was a sort of game; if I got out of the room without waking anyone, I won. Strange things make you happy on nights.

One night I was doing my stealth invader thing when the patient I was trying to medicate suddenly sat bolt upright and said, “Here, this is for you.”

Amazingly, I did not scream or drop the medication.

The young man from Hawaii had come in with a persistent skin infection on one side of his face that had extended into his jawbone. He had been treated several times with oral antibiotics with no effect, so he was now an inpatient getting the “full bore” treatment with IV meds. I had never actually seen his face until that moment. The right side was swollen and disfigured with the infection; it must have hurt. But that didn’t stop his impish grin as he handed me a folded piece of paper.

“I wrote this for you,” he said. “Read it later.”

I forgot about it until I was home cleaning out my uniform pockets. I’m not sure what I thought it would be, but as I read it I had to sit down. This was a love poem and yet not. He was saying how nice it was, in this place, to see someone smile, not at him particularly, just smile. “Wahine (Hawaiian for woman), always smiling” was part of what he wrote.

For the next few nights he was awake for his 2:00 a.m. dose and we had a handful of short, whispered conversations. I hadn’t realized he had been hospitalized several times before for this condition. His positive outlook was quite amazing given how long he had been sick and how little the treatments were doing for him. We were both homesick; me for snow, him for his family back in Hawaii. He was in L.A. for college, tending bar to support himself, and he loved surfing. All this had stopped, of course, when the infection started. No one had any idea how he’d caught it. Yet there was no whining, not a bit of self-pity. He planned on getting better and getting on with his life and couldn’t see the point of wasting energy on a negative outlook.

We talked about my “smiling.” I couldn’t believe anyone

thought I was smiling all the time. “But you do,” he said. “You smile at the guy when you put up his medication. You smile when you take it down. You smile when you come in at 6:00 to take our temperatures. No one else smiles here. They act like they hate being here and taking care of us is a nuisance. But you always smile. You must love your job.”

I had to leave because I was crying.

I was off for a couple of days and when I came back he was gone, discharged, I supposed. A couple of weeks later I bumped into the doctor responsible for my nocturnal poet. I asked him how this patient was doing. It turned out he had been transferred to another hospital where they could give him even stronger drugs for the infection.

I still have that poem. A few times I've dragged it out and reread it when things were particularly tough. I've often wondered if he knew how much he affected my nursing practice, because now, I smile. Boy, do I smile. No matter how tired or out of sorts I feel, when I approach a patient, I nail a smile on my face that would light up a dark room. People actually think I like working nights, twelve-hour shifts, Christmases, through my daughters' birthdays and school concerts. As it turns out, if you can smile about it, it's better already.

~Trish Featherstone

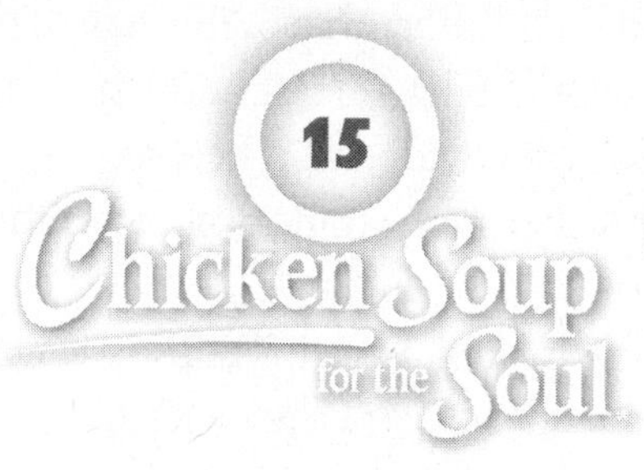

Bobby

Death — the last sleep? No, it is the final awakening.
~Sir Walter Scott

I met Bobby early in my nursing career. I don't remember his specific diagnosis, only that he suffered from a genetic disorder.

I wasn't sure what I would find when assigned to the terminal ward on the pediatric unit that night. I was prepared to be depressed. I looked at the first three empty beds and thought they seemed to relish a temporary respite from sickness and disease. Then I looked at the fourth bed… and my spirit instantly lifted because of Bobby's smile.

A boy held hostage in an aging body, the eleven-year-old looked to be in his seventies. He was three feet tall. "Three feet and one inch," he was later quick to add, "if I really stretch."

Bobby's chest, starting high under his chin and ending at his hips, was shaped like a barrel. His arms and legs looked like toothpicks. His yellow skin was leathery, rough, and wrinkled. Then there was his smile, like a speck of hope shining through the darkness. I couldn't help but smile back.

"I need a bath," he said with a grin as I walked over to his bed. "I have to be clean. I am going home early tomorrow morning to see my brother. I want to be real clean."

I knew from reviewing Bobby's chart that he was not going to be discharged tomorrow or any time soon. As I prepared him for his bath, I gently tried to tell him that. "You have tests and treatments scheduled and those will take at least another week."

Bobby's grin just grew wider, as if keeping a big secret. "I'm going home to see my brother early tomorrow morning," he repeated. "I need to be real clean."

I agreed with the idea of a bath, thinking it would help him rest. And I was glad to spend the extra time with him, to talk and to listen. Knowing he suffered from constant itching due to the poisons building up in his system, I bathed him once and then laughingly bathed him a second time when he kept saying, "Make sure you don't miss a spot. I need to be real clean for tomorrow when I see my brother."

We giggled as I applied lots of lotion. "Okay, Bobby, whatever you say. You are so clean, you squeak. If we put on any more lotion you are going to slide right off your bed onto the floor and get dirty again!"

Bobby did go home. He died shortly after his mother arrived early the next morning. As I comforted her, I told her about our last hours together and the joy he got out of something as simple as a bath. "I'm just sorry he didn't get to see his brother again; he talked about going home to see him."

She looked puzzled as the tears streaked down her face. Then she spoke softly. "I had another son years before Bobby was born and he died at birth. But I never told Bobby. I've never told anyone." She smiled through tears. "But somehow Bobby knew."

~Debbie Sistare

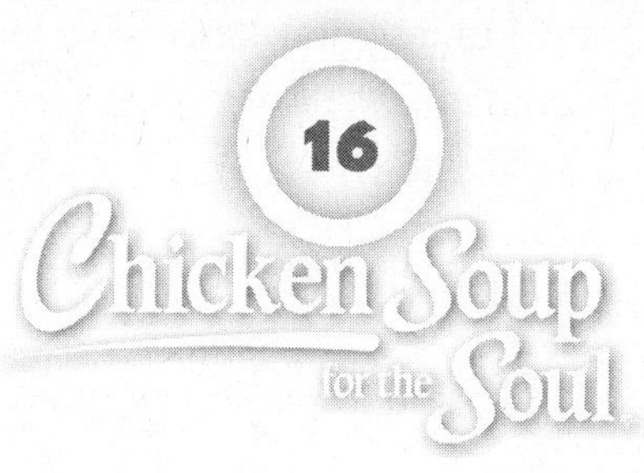

Memories

The joys I have possessed are ever mine; out of reach, behind eternity, hid in the sacred treasures of the past, but blest remembrance brings them hourly back.
~John Dryden

It was the end of my shift, and I pushed open the door to the patient's room to see if any relatives or friends had come to visit. None had. She was such a frail little lady and multiple strokes had left her with difficulty speaking.

I pulled up a chair and sat beside her bed. She did not move. Knowing that she had been an English teacher, I spoke of the influence she must have had over her students through the years.

She did not answer any of my gentle questions. But I sensed she was aware of my presence, so I continued talking about what her days teaching English must have been like. I told her that I remembered vividly one of my English teachers and how I enjoyed poetry at that time.

Still no reaction.

I started quoting Wordsworth's famous poem: "I wandered lonely as a cloud that floats on high o'er vales and hills." I continued reciting the poem, and when almost to the end, I paused.

This sweet lady turned her head and as clear as a bell said, "And then my heart with pleasure fills, and dances with the daffodils."

She fell asleep, and I quietly left her room, humbled by the fact that God gives us memories to retrieve when he feels we need them most.

~Diana Millikan

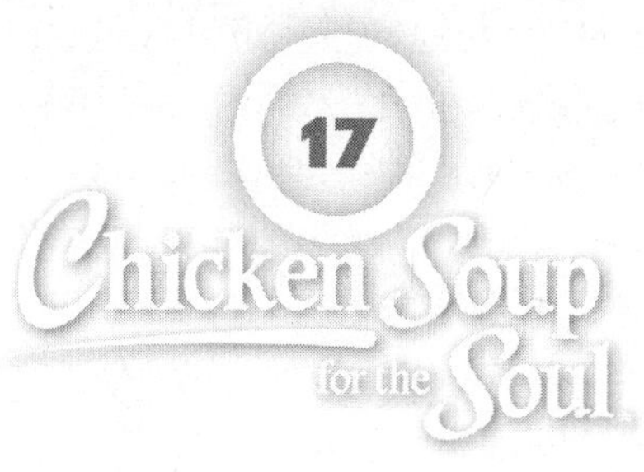

A Better Nurse

The purpose of human life is to serve, and to show compassion and the will to help others.
~Albert Schweitzer

The door closed again, blocking my view of life on the other side. Hot salty tears slid from my eyes. This was the morning of day number three in isolation. IV fluids flowed into my right arm and I was too ill to move. I assumed it was because I was expected to die.

Three days before I'd given birth to my third child, my second son. I saw him for a few minutes and then he was gone, taken away to the nursery while I was wheeled to a different floor. I had not seen my baby since. I had Hepatitis A, probably from drinking contaminated water, the doctor said. He also said I was dying when I was wheeled into the emergency room, but they were going to try to save my baby. That was all I could hope for. Before they could set up the OR for the emergency C-section, I went into spontaneous delivery.

My baby boy was healthy, but I was in grave condition. My liver had sustained so much damage that, even though I'd survived, the outlook was still grim. I tried to shut those thoughts out. I longed to go home with our new baby and mother my children. Breathing was difficult; my head swam.

My condition scared many people. Just to enter my room nurses had to scrub their hands, and then put on a gown, paper shoes, gloves and a mask, and carefully take them off again before they could leave. I felt like a burden to everyone. Few people came into my room, so I had spent the past two days in solitude with the exception of nurses coming to check my vitals and change my IV bags.

"God, please let me just go ahead and die. Anything is better than this." This was not the first time I had prayed that silent prayer. Fighting, it seemed, was futile.

The door opened and a large woman dressed in white walked in. "Good morning, honey. How are you today?" Her strong Southern accent was soothing. As she leaned over me to straighten my pillow, she saw the tears. "Why, sugar, what is the matter with you?"

Unable to speak, I just looked at her. I watched her as she assessed my condition. She checked my face, hands, arms, and then lifted the sheet to check my feet and legs.

"When was the last time you had a bath? And, where is your breakfast tray?"

Embarrassed and confused, I shook my head. "I haven't been able to get out of bed to shower."

"Oh, honey. You don't get out of bed. You get a bed bath. You're too sick to get up, child." She moved around the room as she spoke, bending over and removing a plastic basin from the bedside table, gathering towels and washcloths she'd brought in.

"Did you get breakfast this morning?"

"No. I haven't had food in two days."

"Well, you just wait a minute." She opened the door to the bathroom and returned carrying a basin filled with warm water, soap and shampoo. She pushed the call light hooked to the side of my bed. A nurse's aide came to the door and said, "Yes?"

"You call down to the kitchen and tell them the woman in this room has not received her breakfast and we need it right now." The aide disappeared.

The nurse bent over me, and using the warm washcloth, gently wiped the tears from my face. "Don't you worry, honey. I'm going to give you a bed bath and wash your hair. Then we'll put lotion on you and get you sitting up, and then you will get your breakfast."

"But I thought I wasn't supposed to get anything because I may be dying."

Her eyes widened as she pursed her lips together tightly.

She washed my hair, rinsing it several times with wonderfully warm water. I could not stop my tears as this wonderfully kind woman took such gentle care of me. As she bathed me, I felt myself come alive as a fresh breath entered my soul. Her gentleness and kindness brought me back to life as she ministered to me. She applied lotion to my arms, hands, legs and body. Still, I could not stop crying.

When she finished with her ministrations, I expected her to leave. She surprised me by removing her isolation attire and going out into the hallway to retrieve my lunch tray from which aromas wafted, making my stomach growl.

Gallantly, my angel reentered my room, again completely covered in protective attire. She rolled the head of the bed up, propped me up with pillows, smoothed out my covers, and then fed me. Food had never tasted so good. I still could not stop my tears. Gratitude filled me… filled my heart until I could hardly stand it. She talked to me softly while she spooned the food into my mouth. I will never remember what she talked about and I do not recall what she fed me. But I will never forget how her kindness nurtured me.

Years later, after I graduated from nursing school and went to work, I remembered how it felt to be ignored and how wonderful it was to be cared for with loving kindness. If I take a little longer with my patients, or do a little extra for them, it's because of the gentle woman who showed me such love. I don't know her name, but I will always think of her as the angel who taught me how to be a better nurse.

~Jo Davis

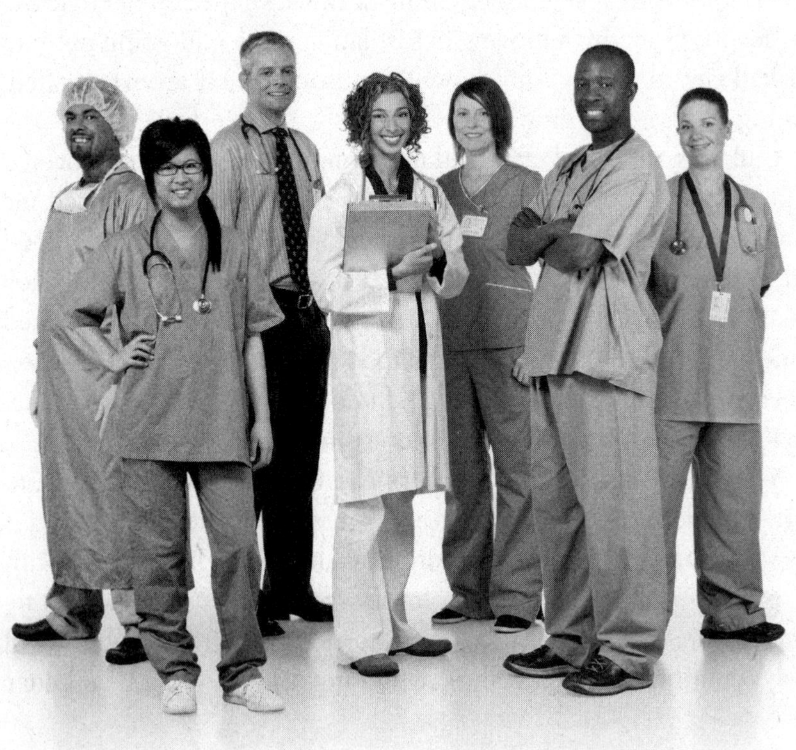

Chapter 3

Inspiration for Nurses

A Calling

If a man loves the labor of his trade, apart from any questions of success or fame, the Gods have called him.

~Robert Louis Stevenson

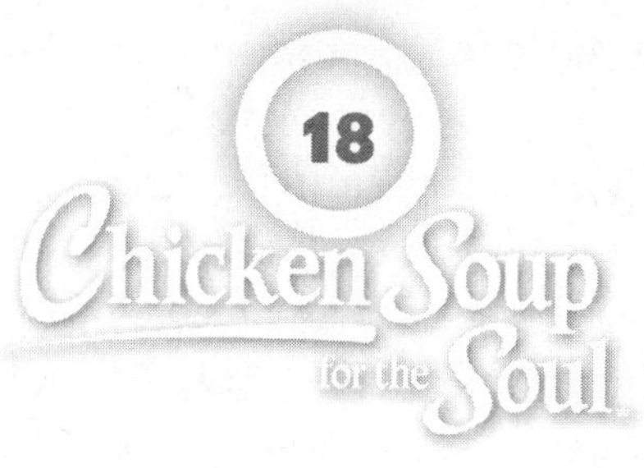

A Nurse Named Mary

The miracle is not that we do this work,
but that we are happy to do it.
~Mother Teresa

We'd prayed for weeks for a miracle as Mom lay dying from liver cancer. When the young woman first appeared on our doorstep, she looked more like a lost hitchhiker or penniless college student than a hospice nurse capable of alleviating Mom's pain. The tall and thin woman at the door slouched forward beneath a backpack slung over her shoulder. Her straight hair was a dull, light brown and pulled back into a ponytail that flipped back and forth when she turned her head.

Even though it was a warm day in January, she wore a blue, knee-length ski jacket over her white uniform, so it wasn't clear at first that she was a nurse.

I reached for the doorknob and pulled the door open.

"I'm Mary," she said, with a directness that was surprising, "the nurse sent to take care of your mother."

Earlier that day someone had called from Mom's oncologist to tell us the doctor was sending a hospice nurse to help us, so we were expecting her. Mom was so sick I could hear her pleading through the walls of her bedroom each night for someone to stop the pain.

Still, I didn't want to let Mary into the house. I knew that once she stepped over the threshold our lives would change forever.

Until the cancer had taken a turn for the worse, my father, brother, and I had been able to take care of Mom. We brought her home from the hospital and gave her aspirin and medicine to help with the pain. We carried cups of hot tea upstairs whenever she was thirsty. And we made sure she had ice packs and heating bags if she needed them. We weren't ready to admit that we could no longer take care of her ourselves. Most of all, we didn't want to hand over her care to a stranger.

So, on the day that Mary appeared at our door, I saw neither a miracle nor an angel. Instead, I saw an intruder, an interloper, a thief who would steal Mom from us rather than someone who might help her better than we could. As her son, I wanted to be the one who read aloud to her from magazines, or comics in the daily newspaper, or from the pages of her favorite books. I wanted to be the one who tuned the radio to her favorite stations. It's what Mom did for us when my brother or I had gotten sick. Mom made us stay home from school and would sit with us in our bedrooms to keep us company, in case we needed anything. Now I wanted to do the same for her.

Mary stood patiently at the front door, waiting to be invited in. How I dreaded the sight of her walking through the doorway.

After leading Mary upstairs to Mom's bedroom, I watched as she sat on the bed and introduced herself. The moment they met, it felt as if Mom's body relaxed, as if she had re-discovered a long-lost friend, a soul mate, after years of separation. From that moment on, Mom confided to Mary all of her fears and worries, all of her dashed hopes and dreams.

I can still see the two of them in the bedroom: Mom's head pressed close to Mary's, the two of them whispering secrets, giggling and laughing like schoolgirls, Mom sharing secrets with Mary (secrets I'll never know) while Mary's long, thin arms wrapped themselves around Mom's shoulders, hugging her as she rocked her to keep the pain at bay after the powerful drugs had worn off and before it was time for her next dose.

Every day Mary brought Mom a measure of comfort that was impossible for my brother, my father, or me to give her. What Mary brought her was the truth. She spoke to Mom about dying without hiding anything from her, unlike Dad, who had wanted to shield Mom from pain and disappointment. Perhaps he was afraid the truth might be too much for her to bear. Or perhaps he simply couldn't bear it himself.

If anyone had asked me then to write our family's motto on a flag to proclaim our cause, it would have read: "Keep fighting, Mom!" Dad was convinced if we encouraged Mom to keep fighting, she would get better. And I believed him. If Mom could fight long and hard enough, I told myself, she would persevere and win back her health.

But Mary knew the truth of cancer better than any of us. As a hospice nurse, she knew how sharing the truth could give a patient the strength to face reality. The way she revealed the truth to Mom, gently feeding it to her with the utmost care and love, the way you might spoon-feed an infant, helped make Mom's journey into the unknown easier to bear, less bewildering, less frightening.

As Mom's strength waned each day and the pain grew more intense, Mary became her best friend, her confidante, her co-conspirator. She stayed with Mom practically every moment, rarely leaving her bedside. During those days I watched her dispense medicine for pain and give Mom back rubs and foot massages. I wished I could have done that, but I didn't how or what to do.

Without Mary, the last days of Mom's life would have been an agonizing journey into the unknown, alone. Mary helped make the journey an adventure, a road to share with a friend, a way for Mom to participate fully in her life rather than letting death cut her off from it.

Before Mary knocked on our front door, we had prayed for a miracle to save Mom. We hadn't realized that Mary was the miracle we actually needed.

~Bruce Black

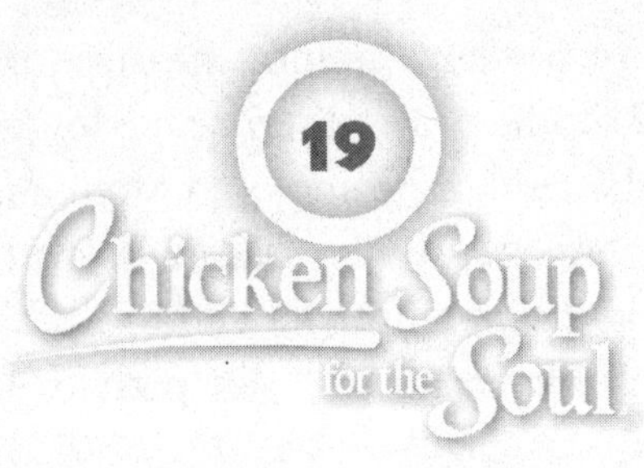

Living the Dream

I know the plans I have for you.
~Jeremiah 29:11

My dream haunted me as I pondered the details. I saw hallways, metal louvered doors, desks, test papers, and just before waking, I felt the strong impression I needed to return to school. But in reality, that didn't make sense. It actually seemed outlandish. I was a wife and a mother of three rambunctious boys, ages five and under.

I'd become pregnant just before my seventeenth birthday. Back in 1972 a pregnant teenager wasn't encouraged to stay in school. So I married my beau and started a family. Finances were tight and I often wondered if there was some creative way I could bring some extra money into the household. Going back to school was not an option, as it would place a huge strain on our already-tight budget. There was no way we could afford childcare, tuition, books and the other extra expenses.

Going about my daily tasks, I couldn't get that dream out of my mind. Time and again, it recurred, perplexing me.

As I placed a roast in the oven, or folded the laundry, I had that eerie sense I had to return to school. I knew only a small fraction of teenage mothers completed their education; I tried processing what was happening, why I felt this strong urgency to do so.

One afternoon, after putting the boys down for their nap, I took the opportunity to catch a few moments of rest. Sitting in my comfy chair, I drifted off into a half-sleep, only to be abruptly awakened with that lingering thought: "I have to go back to school."

"That's it," I said. "I need to seriously think about this." As I entertained the possibility, I wondered, "What career would I choose?"

Each day I picked up a paper at the local newsstand and scoured the want ads to see what careers were in demand. I looked over maid and waitress positions. No thanks. I had plenty of that at home. Besides, those jobs didn't require a college degree.

I thought about teaching a health class, but a teaching degree, with its internships and student teaching requirements, would take too long.

As I searched the columns of job postings, time and again, nursing ads caught my attention. I liked the various opportunities available to nurses, the pay, and the idea I could work part-time and still be there for my three boys. I'd had an interest in pregnancy and childbirth since my fifth grade science fair project, when I did a display of clay models of fetal development. I won first place and got my picture in the paper.

It started becoming clear to me. I liked everything about becoming a nurse in the field of maternal/child health. The more I pondered the idea, the more it felt like my dream was leading me to my life's purpose.

But it was still just an impossible dream. Until one day, while visiting my mother who lived close by, I casually mentioned, "I'm thinking it would be nice to return to school and get a nursing degree."

Her response absolutely stunned me. "I'm going to be quitting my job soon. I could watch the boys for you."

I contacted our junior college. With plans to take my GED test, obtaining a student loan, and my mother's generous offer to watch the boys, my dream was in motion!

Four years later, I walked across the stage proudly wearing my white cap and uniform. It was surreal as the Director of Nursing placed the tiny silver pin on my collar signifying I was officially a nurse.

Later that night I placed my head on my pillow and drifted off into a sound sleep. It was the beginning of many to come, as I was no longer haunted by that recurring dream. Now I was living the dream.

~Annettee Budzban

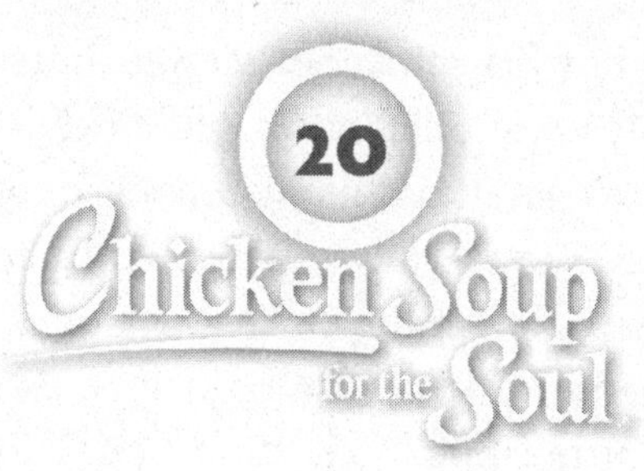

Men Needed

There is no greater calling than to serve your fellow men. There is no greater contribution than to help the weak. There is no greater satisfaction than to have done it well.
~Walter Reuther

In the spring of 1971, a lead story in Sunday's newspaper magazine read "Men Needed." The article reported that nursing was opening up to men and there would be a great demand for them in the future. My husband Larry had recently been honorably discharged from the Air Force and was attending college on the GI Bill. Civil engineering was his field of study, but he wondered if there might be another career for him.

"Look at this." Larry pointed to the article. "I should look into becoming a nurse."

"But you can't even stand the sight of blood. Your hands got clammy and you almost fainted watching a film on chest surgery in our personal hygiene class," I reminded him.

Although he had never considered nursing or any other medical career before that moment, the next day he called the local city college and asked about the process for acceptance into the nursing program.

After completing the application and interview, Larry could hardly wait to tell his family his plan to be a registered nurse. Unfortunately neither his father nor his stepfather viewed nursing as a career for men. Larry was steadfast. "I'm supposed to do this." He said. But just in case he didn't get into nursing school, he also applied for the California Highway Patrol. He was accepted to both programs, and he chose nursing over law enforcement.

Larry graduated in 1974 with his degree as an RN. He would spend his career in rehabilitation, education, and the cardiac catheterization lab, but his real stories took place when he was off duty. Larry always seemed to be "there" when people needed him.

He was still in school when a young boy cut his head badly on a travel trailer where we were camping. The blood would not stop spurting so Larry used his fingers to hold pressure on the wound while the boy's dad drove to the nearest hospital.

One Christmas night a neighbor pounded on our door. A guest was having a heart attack. Larry started CPR and waited for the paramedics. "She won't make it," he told me when he returned home. But two weeks later, she came to our door with a two-pound box of candy to thank Larry for saving her life.

He was "there" again when he saw a young girl fall off the playground bars. The bones in her arm protruded. Larry stopped her father from scooping her up in his arms, thus averting more damage. He used thick pieces of cardboard to stabilize the fractured arm during transport by a private vehicle to the hospital.

Sitting on a tram at the Grand Canyon, he heard on the radio that someone was having a heart attack at the next stop. He asked the location of the person and approached the scene, then took charge of the situation until help arrived.

Once when waiting to be seated in a restaurant, he saw two men dragging a woman out toward the entrance. He approached the trio and asked, "What's wrong?"

"She is having a diabetic attack and we need to get her home."

"She's not going anywhere," Larry cautioned. "Penny, call 911," he directed me. "This lady will die before she gets home." He asked a waitress for syrup, which he had the woman drink.

Then a family on a snow trip had an accident when their sled turned over on a downhill slope. Five people were ejected and one young woman was badly hurt. Larry quickly assessed the situation while waiting for help to arrive. He asked for my sweatshirt and wrapped it around the woman's neck to stabilize it. Once the paramedics arrived they cut my sweatshirt off her and used their equipment to stabilize and transport her to the hospital. Two months later, she found Larry at the hospital where he worked and gave him flowers. "The doctor told me whoever took care of me on the scene of the accident took steps that prevented me from being paralyzed."

Larry held the hand of his stepfather as he struggled in his last minutes of life, telling him, "Relax. Take a deep breath. Go on to Jesus." The calmness of his voice allowed his stepdad to let go of this world.

The most poignant off-duty nursing was when Larry spent hours caring for my brother Sam while he was dying from cancer. Under the direction of hospice, Larry got up every hour to check on Sam and ensure he was pain free, while the rest of the family sat with my brother on two-hour shifts. It was Larry who gathered the family around and held Sam's head as he took his final breath.

These are but a few of the many stories of Larry serving in those unexpected off duty moments. He certainly answered the call… *Men Needed.*

~Penelope Childers

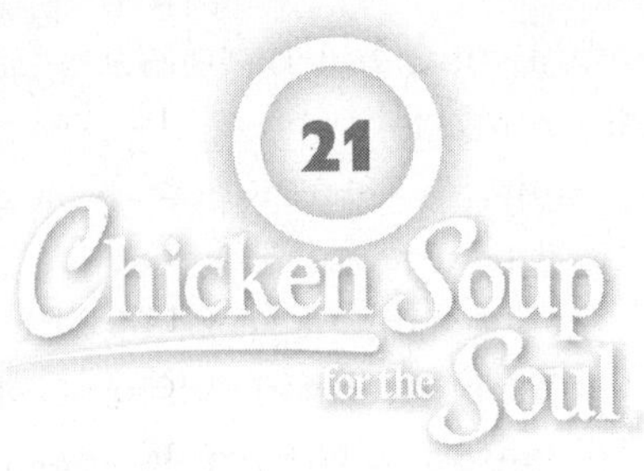

The Spouse of a Nurse

The trained nurse has become one of the great blessings of humanity, taking a place beside the physician and the priest....
~William Osler

The nursing field attracts only the finest individuals. The demands placed on a nurse are not only physical, but emotional and mental as well. These demands are also, to a lesser extent, felt by the family of the nurse.

The parents of a nurse see their child entering a career full of hardships, long hours, and stress but know it is a special calling that only a few can answer. Unbeknownst to the nurse's parents, the pursuit of this career began at an early age when they raised their child to be a caring and empathetic person. As the graduate nurse walks off the stage, they bestow hugs, kisses, support, and assurances that the nurse made the correct career choice.

The spouses of nurses enter into an unknown world, unless they also work in health care. The spouses learn that they will see very little of the nurse on the days the nurse works, and days off are spent trying to rest for the next shift. The nurses arrive home with achy feet, stained uniforms, smelling of others' bodily fluids, and after a quick shower, fall asleep as soon as their heads hit their pillows.

The spouses of nurses also learn that their nurse will sometimes cry for reasons known only to the nurse, and no amount of hugs or kisses will stop the flow of the tears. Many meals will be eaten alone since the nurse's hours are unpredictable; working late becomes routine. The spouses know that their love is the greatest comfort.

The children of a nurse say goodbye early in the morning and may see their parent return home late in the evening, many times after they are in bed. The children learn at an early age that they must sometimes put off their birthday celebrations until the nurse's day off, or that a special event will sometimes be attended by only one parent while the nurse is at work.

The spouse of the nurse explains to their children how important the nurse's job is, and how the nurse eases people's suffering. The children respond that they understand, and they smile and put on a brave face, still wanting their mom or dad with them to celebrate their special day.

After the event the children wait with pictures and stories to share, but as soon as the nurse comes home, they run to greet their parent, forgetting their disappointment, forgetting the pictures and stories, but giving hugs and kisses. To the nurse this affection is also thanks for doing a job that often appears thankless.

After working long, emotional, strenuous hours, the nurses go home to be recharged with love, support, and understanding. Then after a few hours sleep, they return to work to face challenges all over again, feeling strengthened by those who love these angels of mercy.

I am the proud husband of a registered nurse. I am also a former Navy corpsman and a former New York State paramedic. I have seen firsthand what nurses go through every day. I do not know if my wife realizes how special she is and the difference she makes in the lives of people.

I am there to dry her tears, to comfort her, to help her recharge. I am there to give her support, motivation and love. But mostly I am there to say thank you to her… and to you… for following a special calling few can answer.

~Mark Anthony Rosolowski

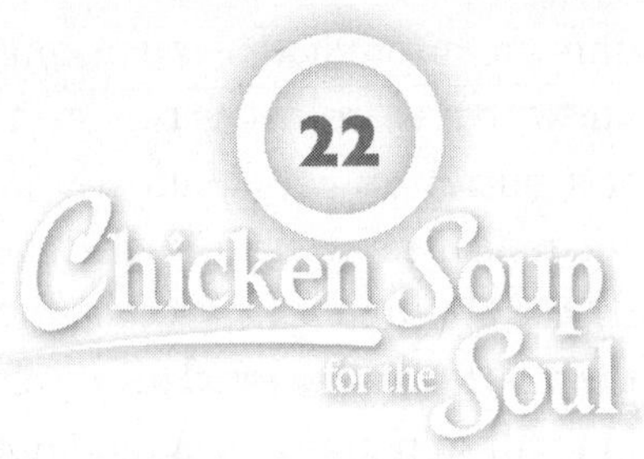

Wait and See

A person often meets his destiny on the road he took to avoid it.
~Jean de La Fontaine

Tears welled up in my eyes as I sat in the Intensive Care waiting room with dear family friends. My deep emotions were not just for the family as they dealt with the life and death issues of their eighteen-year-old, they were for the compassionate nurse who had already "clocked out" but was spending her own time explaining everything she could to this traumatized family. The young patient was caught in that critical place between life and death. No one could tell them for certain what the next day or two would bring. Yet this caring ICU nurse shared her knowledge and experience, educating and preparing the family with honesty and loving kindness.

I quietly observed the beautiful give and take of such a vital conversation between a loving nurse and worried family. It finally seemed as if all that could be said had been discussed, so the nurse stood up to go home to her own family after working all day. I got up to leave with her, for the nurse was my daughter.

It was almost impossible to believe this dedicated nurse was the same little girl who passionately hated germs and sickness. All the way home, my mind was flooded with some of those early memories.

Because of her great dread of germs as a little girl, Chrissy wouldn't even sip a drink after someone else. I suppose her fear was understandable, because for most of her life her dad had been deathly ill from lupus. The constant trauma of infections, hospital stays, ambulances, and emergency and intensive care visits was hard enough for her dad and me to handle; it was extremely challenging for a young girl living under the constant threat of her daddy dying.

During one major crisis, when Chrissy was fourteen years old, she couldn't bear to hear details of the latest catastrophe. All she wanted was a normal teenage life. My husband had "died" and was revived, only to be put on life support for over a month. As I walked with my daughter toward the unit where her dad lay with machines doing everything for him, I tried to prepare her for what she would see. She put her fingers in her ears and sang to keep from hearing the news.

On another occasion, she was so traumatized by the steady barrage of medical emergencies that she blurted out, "When I grow up, I never want to be around sick people!" I was so stunned by the rude remark in front of her dad that I wanted to scold and correct her, but something kept me quiet as she ran off in anger. A little voice quietly whispered to me, "Just wait and see." Though I had no idea what those words meant, I knew I was supposed to remember them.

Chrissy's dad died when she was fifteen years old. She had lots of problems dealing with his illness and death. She married young, became a mom, and lived a lot of life the hard way.

Then one day, a decade later, she announced she was going to college to become a nurse. That was the last thing I thought she would want to study! Even though she made excellent grades all through nursing school, I still shook my head in disbelief every time she talked about what she was learning.

Her dad didn't get to see her enter nursing school and graduate at the top of her class. Or perhaps he did. Maybe he was present as she walked across the stage to become an RN. I believe there are those God calls to be a nurse. My daughter is one of them. She tried to run from it, but she finally gave in and found her place, where she serves with passion.

I am so blessed I got to "wait and see" the beautiful loving nurse God called my daughter to be.

~Eva Juliuson

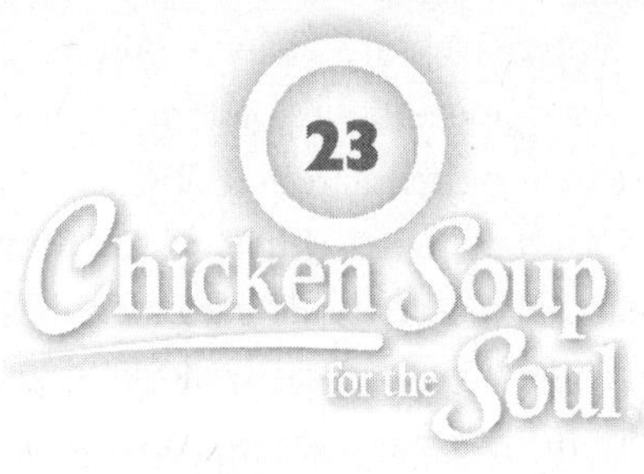

The Invulnerable Child

If you truly believe in the value of life, you care about all of the weakest and most vulnerable members of society.
~Joni Eareckson Tada

The call came in at 2:00 a.m. "Young female runaway needs help."

Police often called from the hospital when they suspected a mental health problem. As a Community Mental Health Nurse, I had spent many nights with students who had overdosed, women who had been abused, and teenagers who'd lived in far too many foster homes. The voice at the other end of the telephone sounded urgent.

Because of the hour, my husband insisted on keeping me company. He was used to driving me on late-night visits. It gave us a chance to catch up on our busy lives.

In the hospital, I was rushed into a private room while my husband settled in the hallway with his book. A tiny girl of seventeen sat on a cot with her back to me. All I could see was her long, matted, vibrant red hair. "Red" turned to face me and my heart melted. I had never seen such a lonely looking child. She reminded me of a doll our girls owned when they were little—Miss No Name.

"But why?" I asked the policeman standing guard.

"We found her huddled in the stairwell of an apartment building, with a weapon. Refuses to pass it over."

"A weapon?"

"A jackknife, curled up in her hand."

Red opened her fist and showed me the little knife. Our eyes met as I passed her a cup of hot chocolate.

Conversation wasn't easy. I had to be patient. We sat for what seemed like hours while my husband kept sending in treats. My role was listening. Red's pain welled up with silence and then guilt. Between hugs, words seeped out, as if crying for release. Eventually, I learned her family had disowned her because of her erratic behavior.

"I get wound up and run the roads," she said. "I can't help myself. I don't know why I do these things. I run and run and don't eat or sleep."

"And now," I asked. "How do you feel now?"

"Exhausted."

"But why the knife?"

"I don't know. I just want the pain to end."

While the policeman hovered close by and Red accepted the doctor's medication for sleep, I thought of my own family and wondered why some children suffered so much. After telephoning several numbers she'd given me, I reached an aunt who offered to help. As I explained the situation, the aunt said she would take Red into her home until she recovered.

"Life hasn't been easy for her or her family," she explained. "My niece was a terrific child when she was young. Kindhearted and loving. Always helping others. But my sister is a single mom now and doesn't know where to turn during the frightening mood swings. There are so many arguments."

I asked the hospital staff to keep Red until the psychiatrist visited in the morning. While the attending doctor and patient advocate scrambled to find a bed for her, I gathered my thoughts and wrote my nursing diagnosis: bipolar disorder, a roller coaster ride with wild highs and devastating lows. Red's symptoms hadn't included hallucinations or delusions, but I still worried. With her persistent feelings of helplessness and hopelessness, I feared she was heading for a major depression, with suicide a serious risk.

I knew what I had to do. I had to protect Red from herself, with education, and most important, with loving care. I promised I would do all I could to help this little girl tackle her illness and the stigma involved. I reminded myself of a quote from the book, *The Invulnerable Child*: "Against all odds, they cope. And they survive." Although there's no cure for bipolar disorder, there is recovery.

By self-managing her medications, the cornerstone of treatment, and with support from family, friends, and self-help groups, Red could one day lead a healthy and productive life. She had already proven she was a survivor. Our journey into wellness had begun.

Several years after our daily, then weekly, then monthly appointments, Red visited me again. She wanted me to meet her husband. And her beautiful red-haired daughter. "And," she said excitedly, "I've been accepted into nursing school and plan on specializing in Mental Health."

As for Red's jackknife. I still have it.

A reminder that against all odds, they cope and survive.

~Phyllis M. Jardine

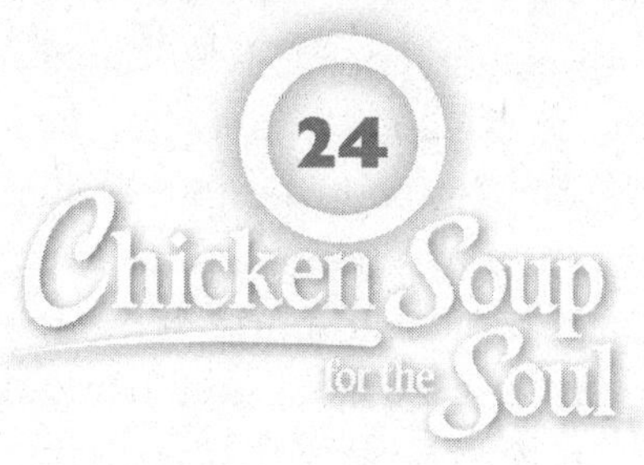

On Call

Wisdom, compassion, and courage are the three universally recognized moral qualities of men.
~Confucius

The phone rings, jarring me out of bed. The digital clock is blinking 2:47 a.m. Already my adrenaline is coursing through my veins. I'm "on call" in the OR so I know who will be on the phone.

We have a gunshot wound of the head, so I need to hurry. I'd laid my clothes beside the bed, ready for just such an event. I pull on my jeans and a sweater, trying to remember where I've left my keys. I kiss my husband hurriedly, hoping he will slip easily back to sleep. He is so used to this routine by now, I wonder if he will realize that I'm gone.

Racing thoughts.

Racing heart.

Racing time.

I start my car. In my mind I'm going over what I'll need to get my team and me through this trauma. I know what instruments are necessary for this case and I mentally go through the list of drugs we will need.

I am capable and ready but my heart beats with tremendous force and speed against my ribs, a rhythm I've grown all too accustomed to. It's the stress factor making me ready for "fight or flight." The ringing phone scared me awake and I'm now in full "fight mode."

I change into scrubs and exit the lounge just as the ER people are wheeling my patient down the hall. The anesthesiologist is "bagging" him and the recovery room nurse is pumping blood. I put on my professional armor, dart past the stretcher and its entourage and hurry to the surgical room. We set the case up quickly, my two nurse colleagues and me, saying little because we know the routine..

As we lift the man to the OR table I notice he is young. Blood mats his hair but the wound on his forehead is small. He is currently stable. Maybe we can save him. The neurosurgeon looks over the X-rays on the view box and then comes to help. The forehead wound is small but is no match for the gaping wound at the back of the head.

Who is he?

Why is he here?

Better not to know…

Suddenly his vital signs become erratic. The scrub nurses stay back, close to the sterile instrument table. The surgeon and I assist the anesthesiologist. The Recovery Room nurse has never stopped pumping blood.

We lost him. Before we've gotten started. I wonder who he was. We stand quietly to take it all in as if we're seeing it for the first time. It seems surreal… the room, the equipment, the young man on the table.

The surgeon goes to the scrub sink and brings back a soapy sponge. Reverently, he washes the blood from the young man's face and hair. He asks for a comb and I bring him one. He combs the young man's hair and says he doesn't want the family to see him until he's ready.

We wrap a fresh, blue towel around his head and I call the medical examiner, as is protocol. I suddenly feel very tired… bone weary… the same sentiment I see reflected in the eyes of my coworkers.

Shortly the young man is on the second leg of his unexpected journey tonight. The OR room is clean… no evidence of the frenzy to save a life. No evidence of the fact that tonight we lost our battle. The room is ready for the next time.

Touched briefly.
A flame burns out.
Will anyone notice?

I drive home more slowly. My husband is sleeping soundly and snoring peacefully. I try to sleep, but can't. There's still the adrenaline. I'm "on call" for two more hours and I need to be ready.

I've put my clothes on the chair beside the bed, just in case the phone rings again.

~Linda Shuping Smith

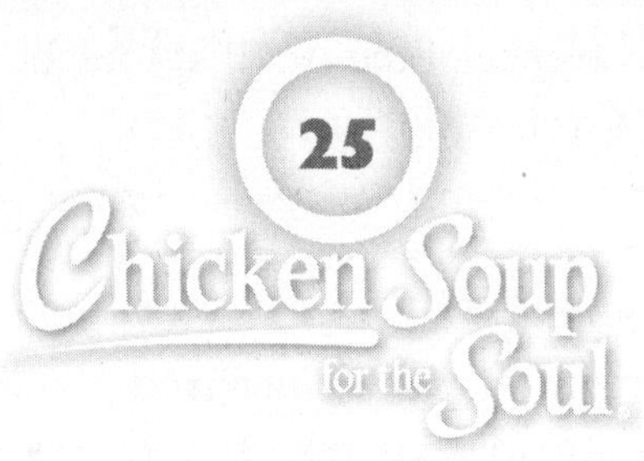

Superheroes

We make a living by what we get,
we make a life by what we give.
~Winston Churchill

Jennifer was a nurse with a loud voice and lots of opinions, which she was more than happy to share with anyone who would listen. She spent many hours in my office lambasting our program and protocols, our agency partners, and anything else she found burdensome and annoying. And she channeled that passion positively as a Sexual Assault Nurse Examiner—a SANE.

A SANE's task is nothing short of heroic. When she is called it means someone has been raped or molested and is experiencing the worst day of his or her life. Many nurses come in after working twelve-hour shifts, often pulled away from their beds in the middle of the night. They leave family events to respond to victims' calls. Part of the job is to build trust and rapport with someone who has been violated in unimaginable ways. She is tasked with asking hundreds of very personal and probing questions and performing full body and, in many cases, genital exams, while attempting to put the victim at ease and giving him or her some modicum of control.

I'd never met anyone who could do this with such grace as Jennifer.

I observed her in action. She had a gift. Professional, approachable, honest and empathetic, she nearly always had her patients chuckling by the end of the exam.

One of my jobs in running the SANE program was to de-brief the nurses after they'd performed cases to make sure they were getting the emotional support they needed to handle the stress of their jobs. One morning I awoke to find Jennifer sobbing on the phone. As often happens with SANE nurses, a well-meaning friend had sent her an article about a horrific child rape in the Midwest.

"People send me articles like this all the time," she cried, "as if I need more trauma." She struggled for a deep breath. "I don't know why this one hit me so hard."

"You just performed an exam last night," I soothed. "Your emotions are raw."

"I've never felt this much rage before," she countered. "How can I have this much anger and still be a good nurse?"

"Besides being a nurse, you are also human," I said. "Feeling outrage over that kind of brutality is normal."

"But I'm supposed to care about people, not despise them."

"Remember the patient you cared for last night? She smiled and thanked you as she left the clinic."

"Right. I admit, we don't get many thank you notes from our victims," she said sarcastically. "We don't see them on the street and get a hug," she added, obviously trying to lighten the mood.

"In your day job you're taking care of people, changing lives, saving lives, and then you shift gears at night to deal with the truly horrendous. You bravely accept the challenges and the consequences, knowing it will weigh heavily on your heart and soul."

"Yes, it does." She took a deep breath.

"Jennifer, your presence in that girl's life last night started her on the way to healing. You helped give her back the control that had been taken away. You were the first step in her recovery."

"Thanks, Amy."

"Jennifer, you and all SANE nurses remind me of the good in the world. Working with you has made me a better person.

"You are a superhero masquerading as an everyday hero."

~Amy Rivers

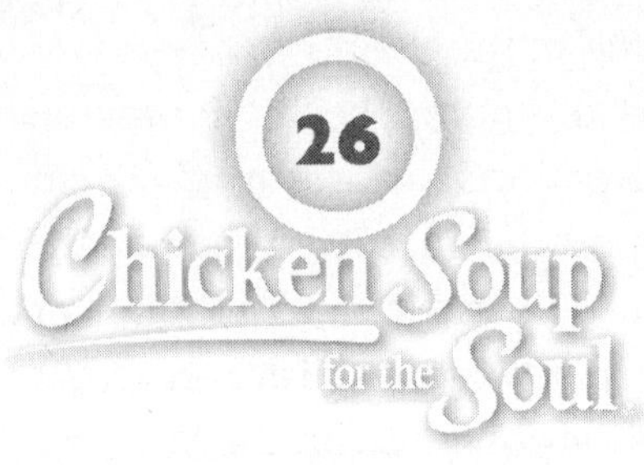

From Hollywood to Healer

If you dream it, you can do it.
~Walt Disney

When I was an adolescent, I dreamed of being a fashion model. I'd grace the pages of stylish magazines, appear in TV commercials and be an actress in Hollywood, too!

A modeling agent in Toronto told my mother, "Annette will never make it." I saw that woman as a dream stealer. I was fourteen years old and, like most teenagers would, I refused to listen. I convinced my mother to let me take a modeling course. Later, I went to see a different agent who decided to give me a chance. Defying the odds, I began to get work and get paid.

By the time I was in my twenties, Toronto was too small for my ambitions. I pursued my dream and headed to Hollywood. A famous agency, Wilhelmina Models, gave me a shot. They sent me out on auditions and I got steady work. I studied acting at the legendary Actors Studio in Hollywood, where stars like Marilyn Monroe, Robert De Niro and Marlon Brando learned. I was cast in numerous small parts in films and was directed by Francis Ford Coppola, famous for *The Godfather*.

I went to film premieres in snazzy movie theaters with famous actors and enjoyed champagne and fancy food at the after-premiere bashes with stars like Paul Newman and Barbara Streisand.

Even with all the glamour and success, Hollywood and the world of fame and fortune left me feeling shallow and unfulfilled. Ever since I was a child, I'd been fascinated by mysticism. I knew early on I had a calling; I was a seeker of wisdom and truth. Yet, L.A. was not nurturing my soul. I didn't go to places of worship nor did I practice spiritual techniques to help me with my suffering. I didn't know what to do.

After several years, I left L.A. and the Hollywood dream. I made my way to Montréal, where I continued my modeling career. I met Gaetano, a handsome, talented artist and sexy French Canadian. We had a whirlwind romance and I became pregnant within the first year of our dating. We joyfully announced the good news to our families. It was the beginning of a long period of shattering heartbreak.

In 1984, I gave birth to Julian, the perfect baby. He never cried or fussed. In fact, he didn't do much of anything. Julian showed zero interest in toys and avoided eye contact. My gut told me there was something wrong, but no one listened. Finally, when he was two-and-a-half, we took him for an evaluation at a local children's hospital.

We got the devastating news. Julian was severely autistic. He also suffered from partial cerebral palsy.

Autism. Cerebral Palsy. It was the start of my dark night of the soul. As Julian got older, unable to talk or achieve independent skills, he became increasingly aggressive. He was considered low functioning on the autism spectrum. He was still pooping his pants at the age of nine, and by that time I was like a zombie, the walking dead. Gaetano and I fought morning, noon and night as our boy flew more and more out of control. We crashed and burned, ending up on welfare — isolated and devastated.

Miraculously, I mustered a little bit of energy. I had contacts in the fashion world and became a buyer for prominent women's clothing lines from Europe. I made good money and we got off welfare but

I was still distraught. I discovered a yoga studio, only steps from my workplace. The classes were a salve to my wounded heart and weary soul, giving me the wisdom and truth I'd been seeking my whole life.

It was there, in the yoga studio, I dreamed of one day being a yoga teacher. I could teach others who were suffering, and help them discover the healing power of yoga. I began to shift from despair and hopelessness to a new inner state of optimism.

Although my inner life was improving, the outer life with Julian and his father continued to disintegrate. Gaetano and I split up. We took turns caring for Julian, who became impossibly aggressive until the day, when he was fourteen, we made the heartbreaking decision to place him in a small institution. It was excruciatingly painful. Every day I was tortured with guilt. It was then, desperate to heal, that I made a bold move.

At age forty-three, I took yoga teacher training at the Kripalu Center in Massachusetts. That changed the course of my life. I began to face my pain stories. I started to meditate and forgive myself, melting my guilt and self-hatred over not being able to take care of my son.

Two years later, I studied with Dr. Deepak Chopra. The training was packed with doctors, nurses and healthcare professionals eager to learn how quantum physics, medicine, yoga and meditation could all be integrated. I envied the nurses who were studying with me and thought, "Wow, what if I was a yoga teacher *and* a nurse? Imagine how many more people I could reach and help."

And so it came to pass. At the age of forty-eight I went to college, and graduated *cum laude* the age of fifty-one as a registered nurse.

Julian is now in a small group home and is surrounded by love. Although he still can't talk, he has learned other communication skills and rarely displays aggression.

During my final year in nursing school, I'd been recruited by a nursing agency to work at a small hospital. I accepted the job, and it was there that my yoga teaching and nursing practices finally merged. Numerous nurses, excited about my methods, inspired my creating and founding the new field of YogaNursing®.

Today I'm creating a global army of modern nightingales, Yoga Nurses, to expand consciousness in health care, relieve stress, anxiety, pain, and suffering for nurses, and improve patient care worldwide.

It's a long way from my life in Hollywood, but it is my dream come true.

~Annette Tersigni

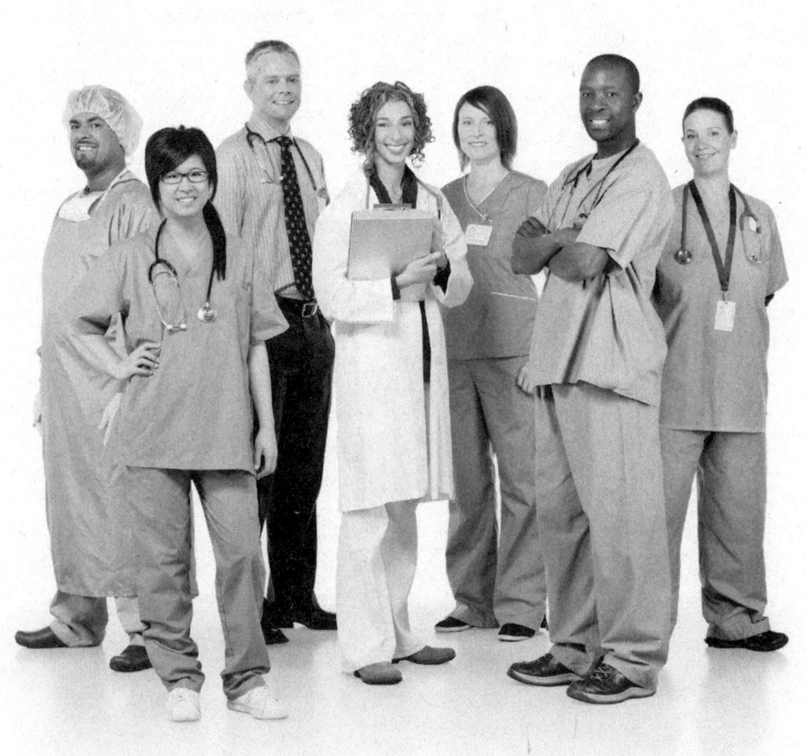

Inspiration for Nurses

Lessons

Life is a succession of lessons which must be lived to be understood.

~Helen Keller

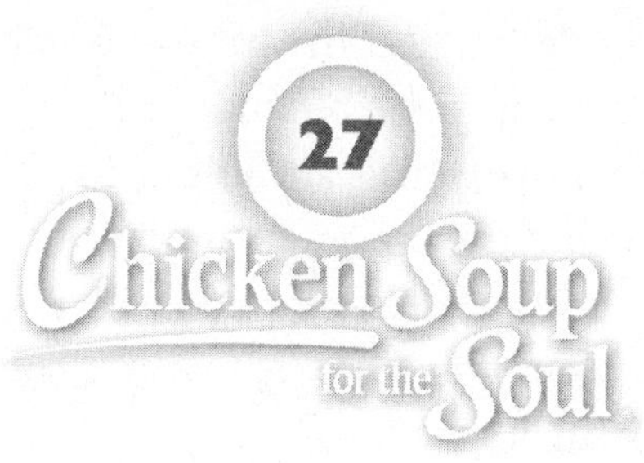

Quiet Refuge

A kind gesture can reach a wound that only compassion can heal.
~Steve Maraboli

Alone in a hospital bed in Baton Rouge, I lay in a cocoon of plaster restraining my body in the hope of repairing my shattered bones. My hospital room was a quiet refuge from the physical and emotional trauma I had suffered at the hands of a rival biker gang. I was a victim in a violent gang war, enduring intense pain after being shot in my left arm and right leg with M-16 rifles.

The body cast encased my left arm, chest, right leg to my ankle, and left thigh. A wooden pole separated my legs. Periodically, I was flipped onto my stomach, exposing a gaping cutout in the plaster necessary for bodily eliminations. Along with the physical pain, the agony of humiliation filled my soul with sorrow and shame.

As I lay in the bed, it occurred to me that I could not find an escape from the uncertainty of the future. My husband, Viggo, had dropped me off at a hospital out of state and left me there, alone and totally dependent on the nursing staff to take care of me. I did not know a soul. That is until Reni, a young nursing student with a reassuring smile, opened the door and stepped inside my hospital room. Her unexpected visit was a welcome relief from my loneliness.

Reni looked beyond the biker girl and we found lots to talk about in spite of our differences. She was pregnant with her first child, and much to my delight, let me feel the baby's movements. Selflessly, she spent time with me, on duty and off duty.

She took care of my personal care needs and frequently washed and styled my hair, which did wonders for my mood. We laughed as she shaved the only part of my leg not covered with plaster. Daily, I became dependent on the life-giving support that her comforting hands and benevolent heart brought me.

Reni stayed with me through difficult physical therapy sessions, holding my hand and encouraging me to press on in spite of the pain. When it came time for the doctor to cut off my body cast, she was there. What a glorious feeling to be free from all that plaster! The months in the cast left my legs weak and feeble, chapped and hairy. She pampered me with the tedious tasks of shaving my legs and massaging cream to restore my skin. Spa treatment in a hospital bed—it felt wonderful.

Yet I faced another surgery. The bones in my leg would be fused together using a bone fragment from my hip. Reni was there when I woke, doing her best to make me comfortable while monitoring my condition. The doctor hadn't mentioned that the surgery would leave my leg two inches shorter. We grieved together over my loss, and her caring spirit helped diminish the pain.

Eventually my father drove from New Jersey to transfer me to a hospital near home. Reni was there in the hospital parking lot, waiting with love and goodbye hugs. It was the last time I saw her, but we promised to stay in touch.

This incredible student nurse, then friend, continued to give me the gifts of compassion and kindness I'd not known from anyone else in my life. Long distance, she inspired me to be strong during the many years of rehabilitation and recovery, plus many more surgeries and hospitalizations.

Today, I have a wonderful husband and two daughters who love me in spite of my disabilities and my past. My passion lies in sharing the message of God's hope and healing for the brokenhearted. As Reni taught me, the power in those acts of benevolence restores our strength… and the results can last a lifetime.

~Maureen Hager

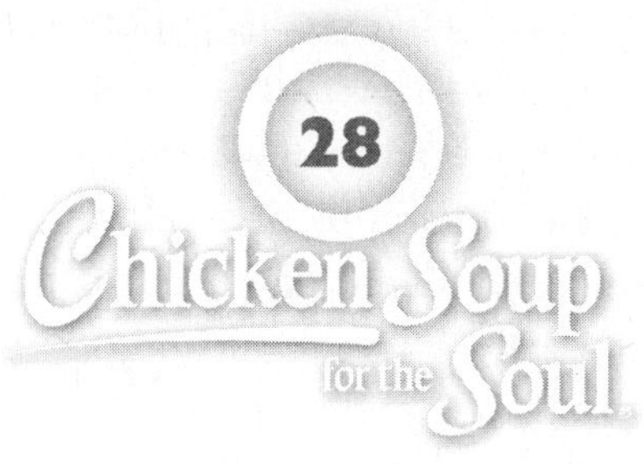

Spring Surprise

The only thing that should surprise us is that there are still some things that can surprise us.
~François de La Rochefoucauld

I was excited about the upcoming obstetrics rotation my junior year of nursing school. My classmates and I considered OB the "happy place" to work. I had the distinct advantage of having three small siblings at home. Many times I had taken my turn at feeding late-night bottles, changing diapers and preparing formula.

According to friends who had completed the rotation, I would likely spend much of my time teaching mothers how to bathe their newborns, using a doll that never cried, wet or spit up formula, and passing out nutritious treats in the sunny kitchen.

True, the actual delivery could be dramatic, but I had already observed a delivery and had successfully squelched the memories of cries coming from the labor rooms.

When a late spring snowstorm arrived unannounced by the weatherman, I eagerly asked for OB when an instructor informed us that students would fill in for staff personnel stranded at home. Armed with the bravado of a nineteen-year-old and my vast personal experience, I believed this undertaking would prove no problem at all.

The unit was nearly empty. Mothers and infants who could be safely discharged had been released.

My assignment was to monitor a patient in the early stages of labor who had arrived when the storm had intensified. I was to report progress to the only nurse on duty, a woman who had already worked fourteen hours and had little hope of relief in the near future.

Before I entered the room I heard my patient scream, "I want Demerol!" I found a Trilene nebulizer lying on the floor beside the bed.

"Here, breathe some of this to take the edge off the pain," I said, beaming my most winning smile.

I ducked as she hurled the apparatus in my direction and yelled, "That stuff doesn't work and it burns my nose!"

Green as I was, even I knew better than to contradict a woman in labor. I certainly was not about to tell her that she had another hour to go before I could dispense more pain medicine.

Her husband murmured soothing nonsense to his wife. The nurse had mentioned earlier that after having three boys, they hoped this baby was a girl.

Stalling for time, I said, "I'll check when you can have your next dose of pain medicine and be right back." I remembered she had a medicine for nausea that might do in a pinch. I explained the dilemma to her doctor when I met him in the hallway.

She was quieter when we entered the room. "You are progressing really well," he said, pleasantly. "Let's hold off on any more medication."

He leaned over her to check fetal heart tones. With energy I never suspected, she sat straight up in bed and nearly jerked the doctor off his feet, grabbing the front of his scrub shirt. Pens and pocket paraphernalia flew in all directions. "Get me Demerol, now!" she seethed through clenched teeth.

Her husband dived for her hands while I plastered myself against the wall trying to regain my wits. The doctor shook himself loose seconds before her right fist connected with her husband's chin. I dashed over with a wet washcloth while the doctor assisted the dazed man into a chair.

Both spouses slept after I administered the injection of Demerol.

"I didn't expect that kind of ruckus," I explained to the seasoned nurse as I charted.

She grinned at my naïveté. "OB is full of surprises. Get something to eat now. I'll probably see you tomorrow." The corners of her mouth drooped as we watched the wind whip up the snow piling higher outside the window.

School regulations allowed junior students to work no longer than eight hours at a time. The next morning I learned my patient had delivered a healthy girl named April Snow.

I paused in the doorway of her room to drink in the scene before me. Mom was bathed, wearing a fresh gown, and cooing at the bundle in her husband's arms. Daddy, with a horrendous bruise on his chin and stars in his eyes, was holding the answer to his prayers.

I understood then that OB was truly the "happy place" filled with surprises. I also understood that, although I might have had vast personal experience in caring for infants, I had a lot to learn about laboring moms!

~Mariah Julio

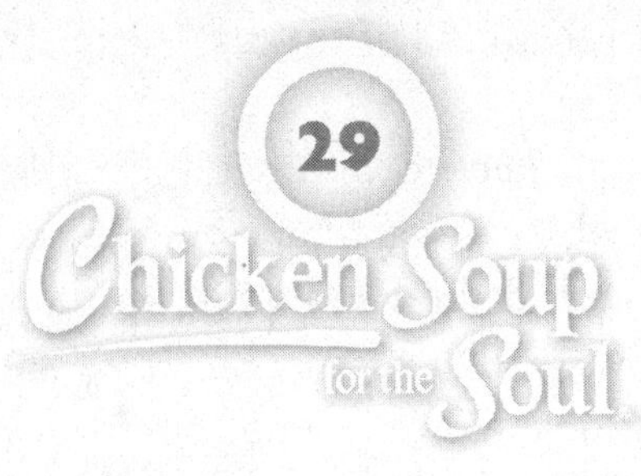

Patients Are a Virtue!

He deserves paradise who makes his companions laugh.
~The Koran

Many years ago a middle-aged man named Bill was admitted to our Med-Surg unit for stomach ulcers. And there Bill was assigned a roommate who drove him nuts.

The college-age kid was quite the chatterbox. He had broken his leg in a motorcycle accident and was confined to his hospital bed with his leg in a cast. He stayed up until the wee hours of the morning, watching television and talking on the phone. Bill would start to drift off to sleep when his roommate's raucous laughter would jolt him awake. This went on for several days.

Sleep-deprived and grumpy, Bill was at his wit's end.

Halfway through his hospital stay, I was assigned a freshman nursing student to shadow me for part of my shift. It was her first day in a clinical setting. When I asked her to obtain a set of vital signs from Bill's roommate, she took his temperature and pulse but hesitated with the blood pressure cuff. "I'm sorry," she said sheepishly. "I don't know how to take a blood pressure yet."

I started to demonstrate how to do so when Bill piped up from behind the privacy curtain. "Just wrap it around his neck and pump up that little black bulb until he turns blue."

~Cheryll Snow

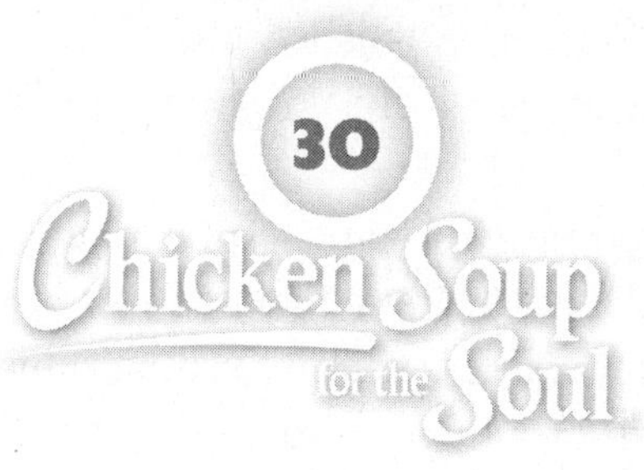

Fishing for Help

True teaching is only achieved by example.
~Plato

Halfway through my nurses training, I worried that I would never graduate. The surgery rotation became my downfall. When I stepped into the operating room, total panic overwhelmed me. My hands trembled and I dropped pieces of equipment. My clumsiness made the surgeons irritable. If a doctor grumbled or criticized me, I became even more flustered. Even my legs betrayed me and I had difficulty standing still. The surgical mask could not hide my teary eyes and red face. The pressure felt so unbearable that I wanted to quit the nursing program and forget my dreams of being an RN.

As soon as I had a day off from surgery, classes, and studying, I made the two-hour bus ride to see my parents. I wanted nothing more than to crash on the sofa and hear words of comfort and sympathy to lessen my stress. Instead, Dad said, "Get moving. We are going to take you fishing." A fishing trip was not what I had in mind for rest and relaxation.

My parents loved to fish, but I had only tried once and had quit from boredom. Without giving me a chance to protest, Dad loaded the gear while Mom packed enough food to stock a grocery store.

My parents launched their motorboat into Lake Winneconne and Dad glided to his special spot on the lake. "This is where the white bass bite," he announced. I relished Mom's freshly caught fish fried into crispy delicacies, but I did not know a white bass from a blue whale.

"All you gotta do is bait your hook with a worm and toss in the line," Dad advised. "With a little practice you will get the hang of it."

I had as much confidence in my fishing skills as being a surgical scrub nurse, which meant zip, zero, zilch. The first worm I squished onto the hook fell off as soon as it hit the water.

"If the worm falls off, grab another and try again," Dad said. I mutilated a few more slimy creatures, but finally maneuvered the worm onto the hook and tossed the line into the water.

"Now keep your eye on the bobber," Dad instructed.

A few minutes passed and Mom hauled in a fish. "Yep, they're biting," she said.

Then Dad reeled in a fish, then another.

I stared into the lake and wondered if I would fail at fishing, too. Suddenly I saw my red bobber go under. I felt a tug on the pole and Dad hollered, "Jerk the line!" I gave my pole a quick tug. "Now reel it in." I did. Miraculously, a wiggly fish dangled from the pole. "See what can be accomplished with a little practice," he said. Dad's grin matched my own. The thrill of catching that first fish motivated me to quickly bait a hook and try again.

The white bass gobbled our worms like starving wolves attacking prey. We'd cast in a line and in a flash we had a fish. It reminded me of the cartoons that show fish jumping into the boat. Within two hours we had our limit. The cooler was full, we were exhilarated, and I had completely forgotten about my miserable surgery ordeal.

We got home and Mom taught me how to filet a fish. At first I was awkward with the scaling, slitting, and cleaning. By the time I finished cleaning my share of the pile of fish, I felt almost like an expert. The day proved rewarding. I hadn't dropped my pole, my hands did not shake, and I slit open a fish with the skill of a surgeon handling a scalpel. Well, almost.

I returned to nursing school rejuvenated. The fishing lesson from Dad made a lasting imprint on my brain. I can still hear his message.

"Bait the hook." (Prepare.) "Toss in the line." (If it does not work the first time, try again.) "Keep your eye on the bobber." (Concentrate on the task.) "Pull in the fish." (See it through.) I applied his fishing lessons to my struggles in the surgery rotation and passed. In fact, his advice helped me all through school and I did become an RN.

As my dad said, "All it takes is a little practice." With Dad's coaching, I learned a lesson to last me a lifetime.

~Barbara Brady

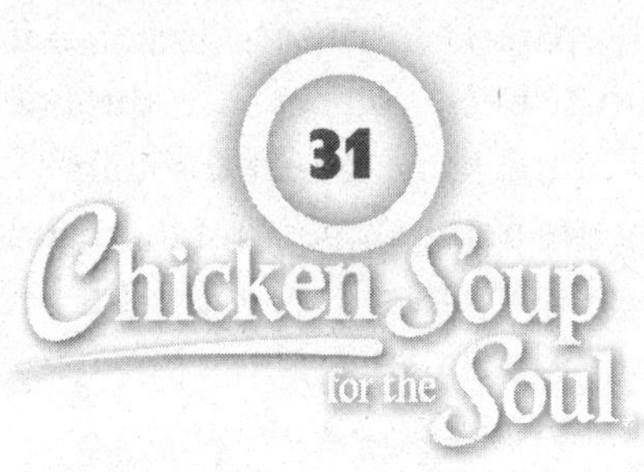

Not ICU!

All truths are easy to understand once they are discovered; the point is to discover them.
~Galileo Galilei

"When did the chest pains start?" the nurse asked. The emergency room buzzed with doctors and nurses scurrying as they hooked me up to various monitors. Part of me felt terrified and the other part too shocked to take it all in.

"We live thirty minutes away," I mindlessly answered, wondering why it mattered. "We left minutes after the pains started."

That afternoon I had felt exhausted, unlike any kind of tired I'd ever experienced. Throughout the day I'd noticed several peculiar symptoms but didn't give them a second thought. I went to bed around midnight. An hour later I awoke, visited the bathroom and went back to bed. According to the clock I'd only slept a few minutes before being jolted from a dead sleep. It felt like cattle were stampeding through my chest. I'd had palpitations before, but nothing like this. I gently nudged my husband awake and told him. "Don't worry," I said, "whatever is going on will hopefully calm down soon."

When I tried to check my heart rate I couldn't find a pulse; my heart raced out of control. I agreed to head for the hospital. My husband grabbed our coats. I kissed our sons goodbye. In the wee hours of the morning, we drove over the state border and down the mountain to our hospital in Woodstock, Virginia.

"Hopefully the medication will convert your heart rhythm and stop the chest pains," the doctor informed us. I threw my worried husband a smile. Once my heart rate had returned to normal, I figured they'd let me go home. But before the doctor left the room he explained I'd be staying in the ICU.

"Why the ICU? Can't she stay in a regular room?" my husband asked the nurse.

"Nope," she answered. "Everyone on this medication gets monitored in the ICU."

When we'd lived out west, I had spent time in what we had referred to as the hospital's hell room—the ICU. The atmosphere reeked of despair; the nurses were cold and indifferent. During my stay, a well-meaning nurse told us that working in the ICU required a "special" kind of person; someone who could remain aloof. She'd claimed it was the only way ICU nurses maintained their sanity. If that was true, we prayed we'd never again find ourselves in another ICU. And yet here we were.

As they wheeled me out of the emergency room I felt sick. "Not ICU," I moaned. "I wish I could go home," I whispered to my husband. "I don't want to spend time surrounded by sickness, death, and ice-cold nurses."

"I wish you could too." He squeezed my hand.

As we approached the ICU, every person we met greeted us with a kind smile or a "hello." I couldn't believe it. When we reached my room, they took great care in getting me comfortably situated. A warmhearted, concerned group of nurses and aides huddled over me. Pure relief washed over my husband's face. He needed to get to work and had hated leaving me. Now he knew I'd be well cared for.

"Call as often as you want," the nurses encouraged him, putting his mind at ease.

Throughout the day these cheerful nurses and aides went about their tasks conversing merrily with each other. There was no doom or gloom. Their soft laughter and light banter filled the atmosphere with a warm, comforting vibe. When they checked on me, they often lingered and chatted. I felt treated like a queen; their attention to me was over the top. When the day drew to a close, I hated to see them go. I felt as if angels, not nurses, had been hovering over me. Instead of the hospital hell room, I'd landed in hospital heaven.

Two nurses checked on me before they left for the day. "Do you have to leave?" I inquired, immediately feeling foolish for asking such a question.

"Get some rest," one of them answered as she took my hand. "We'll see you in the morning."

Through the slit in my drapes, I watched as daylight disappeared. Once visiting hours ended, I felt alone and anxious as I tried to comprehend all that had happened that day. Would life ever be the same? Alone in my room, I prepared myself for the night shift, assuming my day angels were one-of-a kind.

That night, unable to sleep, the most wonderful nurse came into my room. As we talked, I felt as if I'd known her all my life. As I shared my concerns with her, she took the time to listen instead of brushing my fears aside. When the soft pinkish morning glow peeked through my curtains, I said farewell to my night-shift angels.

On the morning they released me, my angels huddled over me like protective mother hens. When my husband picked me up, I had tears in my eyes. Who would ever have thought I'd be teary-eyed at leaving the ICU? I couldn't help myself. I had expected the worst and received the best. I hugged every one of these special souls who had watched over me.

I saw firsthand that working in the ICU does require a special kind of person.

~Jill Burns

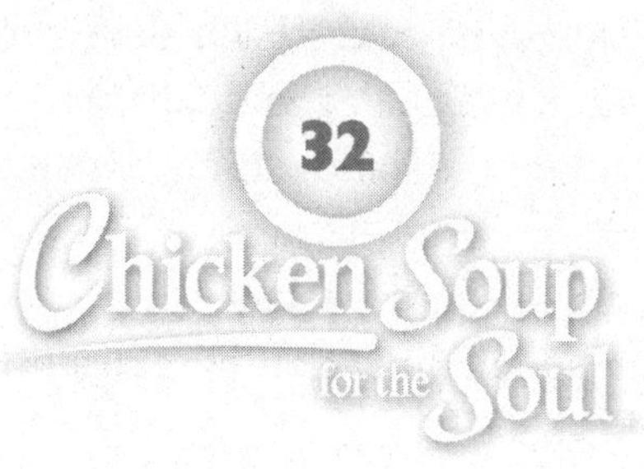

Promises

Promises are only as strong as the person who gives them…
~Stephen Richards

He was sitting in the waiting area of my office with his wife, his eyes red from crying. I shook Kyle's damp hand and asked them to come into my office. As we sat around the table, Kyle held his wife's hand and in tears said, "I am sorry."

I'd had the exciting privilege of assisting in the design and move into our new Midland Memorial Hospital. Yet even more important than creating a state-of-the-art facility with all the bells and whistles was our focus on the staff providing the care. We knew that people being their best provided our patients and their visitors with exceptional care and experiences.

A part of our Culture of Ownership was having every hospital staff member repeat daily the Self-Empowerment Pledge with that day's promise. Monday's promise, for example, was responsibility: *I will take complete responsibility for my health, my happiness, my success, and my life, and will not blame others for my problems and predicaments.* There were promises for each day of the week and we asked our staff to read these together at each change of shift or other times of the day.

Kyle, a registered nurse in our endoscopy unit for many years, was asked by his manager to embrace the Self-Empowerment Pledge and to say it daily out loud with other team members.

Now, through tears, he said, “Each day’s promise was hard for me to say. I went home yesterday and talked to my wife about how conflicted I felt. And then scheduled this appointment with you....” His voice broke.

I handed him a tissue and listened.

“I’ve been doing something that goes against these daily promises... and my own values.”

He went on to tell me that for years he had been diverting narcotics from the unit for his personal use. He was addicted. He assured me that he had never taken anything from his patients. Reading the daily promises had caused tremendous conflict with his values and his actions.

“I’ve been living a lie,” he cried. “I want to get my life back in order.”

He knew there could be serious consequences. He could be arrested for theft. He could lose his job and possibly his nursing license. He could have overdosed or lost his life. The very livelihood he had built for years as a trusted professional nurse was in jeopardy. Completely humbled, he wept, “I’m willing to accept the penalties for my actions.”

Holding back tears myself, I said, “I can’t imagine how much courage it took for you to come talk to me and tell me the truth. I promise I will get you the help you need.”

I followed the steps required by the state board of nursing and the state’s peer assistance program and did everything I could to get Kyle the assistance he needed to heal his mind, body and spirit. He left Midland Memorial for a time and participated in a drug rehab program. Eventually, he reported back to work with stipulations.

As I write this story, Kyle has been 270 days drug free and providing great care to our patients.

I saw him again recently and reminded him, “Kyle, I’m so proud of you and your conviction to right the wrong. How would you even describe this experience?”

“It’s a miracle,” Kyle responded.

By transforming our environment, and focusing on our staff, we keep our promises of exceptional care and witness miracles every day.

~Bob Dent

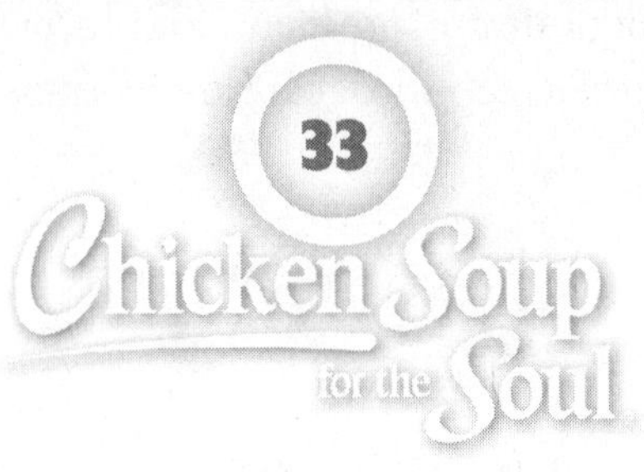

Acceptable Gifts

The greatest gift in life is to be remembered.
~Ken Venturi

One of my home care patients slipped a local restaurant gift card worth $25 into my hand. She told me how grateful she was for my unhurried, careful teaching of self-care for her colostomy. I gently told her, "Thank you so much, but I can't accept gifts."

She protested. "But you took such good care of me, always so patient, repeating everything over and over. I really want you to have it."

Trying not to offend her, I patiently explained that I appreciated the thought, but I was not allowed to accept presents. I was only doing my job. I went on to say, "You have already given me a gift: the gift of courage. Watching you accept your cancer diagnosis, undergo weeks of radiation therapy, then have difficult colostomy surgery, shows me that I can have the courage to stand up to whatever life throws at me."

That incident got me thinking. How many other gifts have my patients given me over the years?

James demonstrated the gift of devotion. He lovingly took care of his wife for several years as her health steadily declined from the ravages of ALS — Lou Gehrig's disease. He learned to bathe, dress, toilet, feed her through a gastrostomy tube, check her blood-sugar levels, and administer her insulin injections. He took over all of the responsibilities of running the household. Their house was always clean and neat, much neater than mine, I have to admit. Well-meaning friends and neighbors encouraged him to place her in a nursing home where she could receive round-the-clock care from multiple caregivers, but he always declined. His devotion to his wife showed me what "for better or for worse" really meant. I came home more appreciative of my husband and his efforts to help with the children and housework after his long day at work.

Will taught me the gift of generosity. He was a community leader, well respected by all who knew him. He lived very modestly although his income was more than adequate. I discovered later that he had given much of his hard-earned money to the local soup kitchen, had established an assisted living facility, and was always there to lend a helping hand to anyone who needed it, all anonymously. Will was a shining example of generosity and altruism.

Brian exemplified the gift of humor. He was my hospice patient, and thus well aware he was dying. At the start of every home visit, he told me a joke, showed me a cartoon, or related a funny story. The louder I laughed, the happier he was. Then I could proceed with the more uncomfortable but necessary treatments I needed to perform. Brian made me realize that humor can be a valuable tool to ease the tension of unpleasant situations. Following Brian's lead, I compiled a file of jokes and cartoons to use with other patients. I thought of Brian every time I dipped into that well-used file of jocularity.

Lauren showed me the gift of dignity. Although she was dying from a prolonged and debilitating terminal illness, she insisted on wearing clean underwear, slips, and stockings every day. She would ambulate painfully over to the sink to hand-wash those "unmentionables" daily. She felt it was undignified if she wasn't fully dressed, with make-up carefully applied, for every visitor that walked through the door, whether it was a neighbor or healthcare provider.

Sue taught me the gift of humility. She was a retired nurse in her late sixties, and I was only in my early thirties. Frankly, at that point in my career I was overconfident. I thought I was pretty knowledgeable about health issues and providing expert health care. My goal of home care was to teach Sue how to manage her new ileostomy. Although her skin was moist and reddened, I showed her the usual way to prepare the skin and apply the adhesive ileostomy appliance. I told her it should last at least until my next scheduled visit three days later. I was disappointed to receive a phone call an hour later that the bag was leaking, necessitating another home visit. We repeated the procedure, and I left to go to my next patient. Less than an hour later, I was called back to Sue's home to replace the leaking bag for a third time. I really was stumped. Sue phoned her daughter, a nursing assistant in a convalescent home, to help us out. Her daughter immediately understood the problem and employed a trick she'd learned: she used a hair dryer to gently dry the skin before applying the bag. Success! I was grateful and very humbled.

The gifts my patients gave me were more valuable, personally and professionally, than any gift card could be.

~Alice Facente

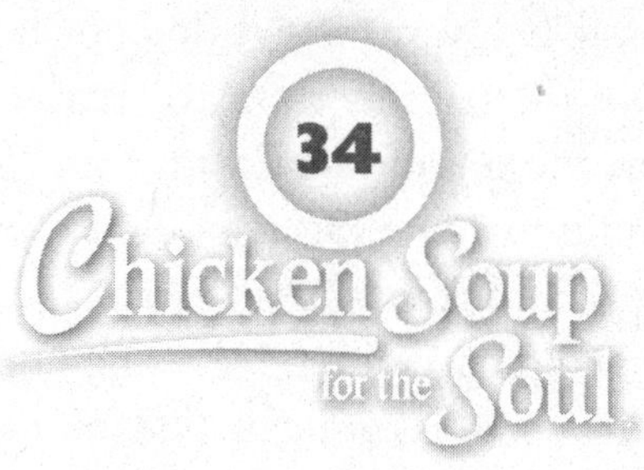

Ms. Picky

It's easy finding reasons why other folks should be patient.
~George Eliot

The day Ms. Picky became the supervisor at the nursing home where I worked as an RN, my secure world crumbled. Of course her name wasn't really Ms. Picky, but her actions fit the label.

I thought I had the perfect job working part-time caring for frail and elderly residents. My nursing career spanned more than thirty years, most of that time as a critical care nurse. I wasn't a novice at dealing with stressful and complex situations. I looked forward to each day at work and felt committed and competent in my job. All that changed when Ms. Picky arrived on the scene.

This new supervisor tackled her duties like a runaway locomotive thundering down the tracks. Nothing fazed her and she made changes immediately. About the time the staff adjusted, she changed procedures again. Then she went on a rampage and fired several nurses and nurse's aides, many without notice or justification. The environment of the facility seethed with tension and hostility. Who would be next to get the axe? For the first time in my life I feared losing my job.

We struggled to make do with a smaller staff. Ms. Picky didn't hesitate to pile on extra duties and then complained if the work wasn't finished according to her timetable. I found myself avoiding her as much as possible. I wasn't above dodging her when I heard her heels clicking down the hallway in my direction. I sometimes even hid in the medicine room until she left my unit.

Attempts to mind my own business, do my job, and avoid conflict did not work. I couldn't manage to escape the wrath of Ms. Picky. It seemed every time I turned around she stood nearby ready to criticize my work or add a new assignment. She found fault and picked at the slightest issues. "Don't fill the tube feeding bags so full. The beds should be elevated 45 degrees. Weigh your patients before breakfast. Empty the trash. Order more oxygen tanks. Write new care plans. Clean the IV stands." Her vocabulary never included "please" and "thank you" nor did she offer a reason for the demands. Not only did she constantly correct my performance, but she did it in front of the residents. I often felt my face redden and my lips quiver as I forced back tears of frustration.

For the first time in my nursing career I was miserable. Every morning before going to work I prayed to get through the day without incurring the wrath of Ms. Picky. In fact, I'd sit in my car in the parking lot and pray again, asking for the strength to endure the criticism and to have the wisdom to somehow satisfy my supervisor. Each day I hoped to survive without being totally humiliated.

Noticing how frazzled I'd become, and tired of my complaints, my husband encouraged me to quit. I had never quit a job and my pride kept me from resigning. Even though I was fed up, I didn't want to give up. Surely I could find a solution to soothe the savage beast in my life.

Obviously Ms. Picky was not a happy person. No one at work liked her and most of us avoided her as much as possible. Admittedly, she worked long hours. A single mom, she often brought her young son to work on the weekends and evenings. I felt sorry for the youngster, who had to amuse himself in her office while she tackled piles of paperwork. I learned she was taking college courses to earn her degree. It became clear that Ms. Picky had monumental pressures.

I knew if I didn't change my approach Ms. Picky would be my downfall. I didn't want to quit my job feeling like a complete failure.

So instead of praying for myself that I would make it through the day, I decided to pray for Ms. Picky. Once I started praying for her my attitude changed. Eventually I didn't even avoid her when she approached. I made myself meet her face to face. Before she could launch into a tirade, I tried my best to pleasantly greet her and inquire about her day, asking about her son and her college classes. I swallowed my pride and even requested her advice on some aspects of patient care.

Ms. Picky gradually shared with me some of her personal problems: her unhappiness about her weight, her struggles with her son, and the adjustment of being in a new city with a new job and no friends. Underneath her tough exterior hid a vulnerable human being.

The more she exposed her inner self, the more likable she became. Much to my surprise, I learned that under her tough exterior she actually had a keen sense of humor. I learned to accept her as a colleague and not an adversary.

I kept praying for Ms. Picky. Before long I found myself once again looking forward to my job. I like to think Ms. Picky mellowed due to my intentional change of attitude. I know my new attitude helped me be more tolerant and less defensive.

Ms. Picky mentioned one day that she had finished her college courses and would receive her degree. Guess who threw her a big graduation party? I did. Not only was Ms. Picky overwhelmed to see the staff gathered in her honor, she entered into the spirit of the party like a friend not a foe. She hadn't yet earned the title of "Ms. Laidback" but "Ms. Less Judgmental" fit.

On that day I celebrated more than her achievement, I celebrated mine.

~Barbara Brady

Tossed Salad

Laughter is higher than all pain.
~Elbert Hubbard

My ten-year-old daughter had been hospitalized for more than three months with a painful, unknown disease. She could barely eat, and when she did her pain level increased dramatically. Both of us were worried, exhausted, and overwhelmed by all the unanswered questions and the unknown diagnosis. My heart was heavy with concern for my beloved daughter. She had missed so many events… her birthday, school activities, soccer games. Her smile had gone missing.

She had been such a happy child, always bringing joy to our family. My prayers were frequent, but my hope that she'd laugh again diminished with each passing day, each medical test that revealed nothing, and each treatment that proved incorrect.

A nurse named Henry gave her special attention and helped me decipher what the multiple doctors said. He brought balloons and made them into animals and visited her every chance he could, even when she was not his assigned patient. Although he was unable to make her smile or laugh, her eyes lit up when Henry came in. He seemed as concerned as I was that the doctors could not find the cause of her severe pain. He became a trusted friend and a nurse who gave us the medicine of friendship and compassion. His concern was our balm.

One afternoon, when Henry brought her lunch tray, she refused all of the food, including Jell-O and pudding. Henry, trying to be funny, said, "You should eat a tossed salad because it's St. Patrick's Day and you need your greens." He put the salad bowl on her food table.

When she didn't laugh and turned her head, Henry took the bowl of salad to return it to the tray on her nightstand. But he tripped over the IV pole, and the tossed salad flew up in the air, sending tomatoes, cucumbers, lettuce, and carrots soaring. Most of it landed on her face and shoulders, with some lettuce decorating her IV pole.

My daughter laughed and laughed and laughed. Months of pain seemed to be released as we all joined in laughter, a discharge of bottled up emotions that had weighed heavily upon us.

"I'm sorry." Henry apologized and chuckled as we removed salad from my daughter's beautiful face. But the more he tried, the harder she laughed.

The doctor came in and saw her tossed-salad complexion. He joined in the laughter and asked, "What kind of dressing do you want?" And we laughed some more.

A few days later, the doctor ordered one more test and thankfully, her illness was diagnosed properly with treatments that began the healing process.

Or was it the laughter?

~Malinda Dunlap Fillingim

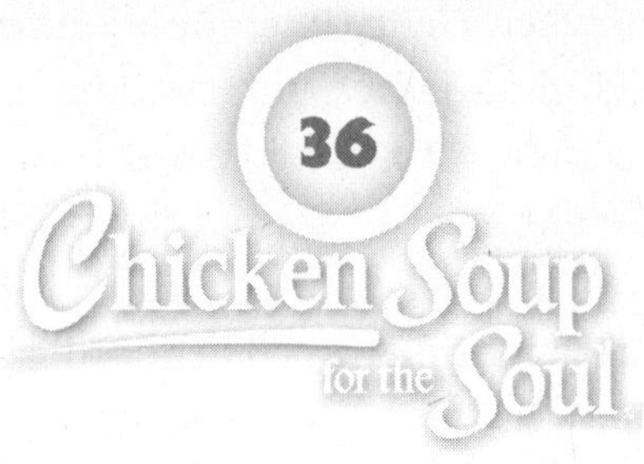

In the Dark

In all troublous events we may find comfort, though it be only in the negative admission that things might have been worse.
~Amelia Barr

"Don't let it close behind you," I warned. Too late. The door clicked shut. With a sinking feeling I realized I was locked in a dark linen closet with Bob, the hospital maintenance man who called me Sweet Pea.

I had just become a registered nurse and this was my second week on the medical-surgical floor of a 100-bed hospital. I'd heard from other nurses that the head nurse, Rhonda, was a terror: demanding, unreasonable. According to legend, she ate new RNs for lunch. But I hoped I'd be such a super-nurse she'd never chew me up. I had successfully avoided confrontations with her so far, but that changed when the closet door locked.

There I was, unable to pass meds and complete procedures, stuck in a tiny dark closet with Bob. Bob, with his slicked-back hair and tight shirts, who patted his round belly and affectionately called it his "beer baby."

I thumped on the door for help but he didn't join in. I pounded harder and began to yell. Finally to my relief, and then horror, I heard, "Who's in there?"

Rhonda. My visions of getting on her good side disappeared into the dark of the room. "It's Carole, your new nurse."

To my further agony, Bob added, "And Bob from Maintenance."

Her voice was granite. "Whatever you're doing in there, come out right now."

In a voice as small as I felt I said, "We can't. We're locked in here." I wondered if she knew the door locked from the outside.

"You're what? Never mind. You should've told me that in the first place. I'll send for Maintenance."

Her heavy footsteps faded and I was alone again. With Bob. Making it worse, I heard him pulling sheets off the closet shelf and plopping them onto what little space there was between us.

"Might as well have a seat, Sweet Pea. This is gonna take a while."

I shook my head. "No, it won't. Maintenance will be here soon."

"Maybe, but it won't do no good. Only one key to this door, and I'm wearing it. Keep telling 'em to get another one made, but they don't listen."

My stomach sank. I wondered if I'd be sane enough to complete who-knows-how-many incident reports when I was finally released.

Just then, I heard footsteps outside the door. I said a silent prayer it was Maintenance and that they'd heeded Bob's recommendation to get another key.

A man's voice boomed. "Bob, you in there with the key?"

"Yep."

There was a pause and then the man said, "Sorry, Rhonda. There's no spare."

Rhonda sounded furious. "You only have one key to this lock?" She called through the door to Bob. "Slip the key under the door and we'll unlock it."

"No can do, ma'am. It's too fat."

With an icy fury, Rhonda said, "Call a locksmith."

"Yes, ma'am. Pronto."

She growled, "Next time, I hope you'll be more efficient."

I was thankful she was talking to the maintenance guy and not me. But my gratitude dissipated along with my deodorant. Minutes seemed like hours and I got hotter in that tiny lightless room where

Bob's too-heavy cologne was giving me a headache.

Bob blew out a deep tobacco-tinged breath and offered, "I can give you a hug if it would make you feel better." Tears formed in my eyes. I was stuck in this linen-filled hellhole and once I got out, I'd probably be fired.

Still wading in my pity pool, I finally heard voices outside the door. Rhonda's was the loudest. "Locksmith's here. Carole, when he gets the door open, I want you at the nurse's station stat."

I had to swallow hard to get my stomach back in its rightful place. "I'll be there."

Once the locksmith opened the closet door, I murmured a quick thanks to my liberators. Without looking back at Bob, I dashed down to the nurse's station on rubbery legs. Rhonda motioned for me to follow her to a vacant room. She closed the door and for a foolish moment I feared she would lock us in.

Words rushed out of my mouth. Apologies toppled over explanations and promises that I'd do better.

She held up her hand for me to stop. "I had to get others to do your job. Our patients couldn't go without their care while you were in hiding."

She made it sound like I'd done it on purpose. I wanted to protest her accusations, but she left me no opening.

She continued. "You haven't been an RN for long and you're new here, but those are not excuses. Everyone's responsible for her actions. And a nurse's actions here are to help patients to the best of her ability." She leaned in toward me and in a low voice added, "I've got my eye on you. Now get back to work."

I managed to hold myself together the rest of the shift, but as soon as I reached my car the tears fell hot and fast down my face. I was sure that Rhonda would find a reason to fire me within the week. I dreaded going back to work.

Arriving at the hospital the following day, I expected Rhonda to watch me like a hawk. Instead of picking apart everything I did, though, she offered suggestions for improving my nursing skills. By the end of the day, I'd learned more than I had in the previous ten days on that floor.

I had my coat on, ready to leave for the day, when I thanked her for her help. She harrumphed. "You're surprised I helped you." She paused and stared at the wall behind me. "I know what everyone says about me. I am tough, but only when I need to be. Even though you did something stupid yesterday, you're a good nurse, not great, but good. Our patients deserve great nurses. And I think you'll get better over time, even if you do need better organization and time management skills."

I didn't know what to say, so I just stood there, my face a blank.

"That's all. Go home."

I rushed to the parking lot but when I got inside my car I just sat and thought about Rhonda. She wasn't really an ogre. She cared about the patients and drove us nurses to provide outstanding care.

It's been a number of years since I've moved past that job, but whenever I'm getting tired, or feeling like I can't provide top-quality care anymore, I remember Rhonda. She inspired me to always do my very best, even in the darkest circumstances.

~Carole Fowkes

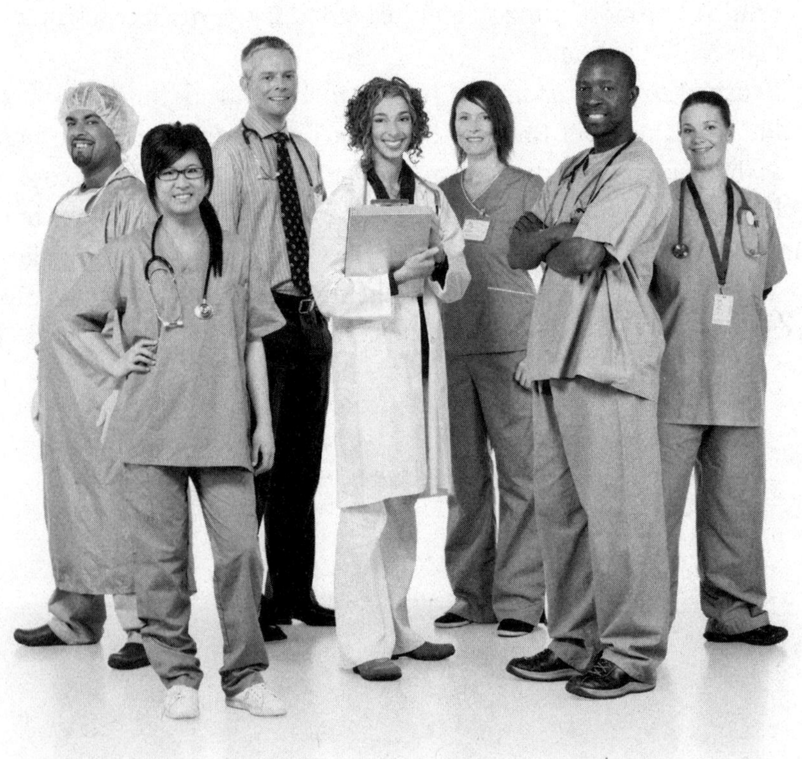

Inspiration for Nurses

Overcoming Obstacles

The only use of an obstacle is to be overcome. All that an obstacle does with brave men is, not to frighten them, but to challenge them.

~Woodrow Wilson

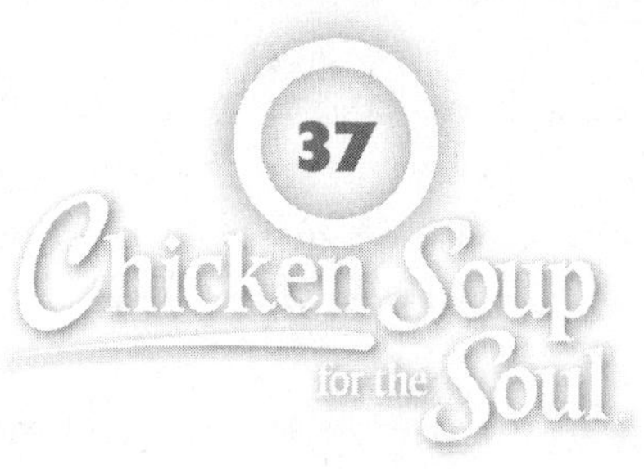

What's Really Bugging You?

I have learned a great deal from listening carefully.
~Ernest Hemingway

As a home health nurse, I frequently find myself doing tasks that are outside the usual scope of nursing practice. I have cooked meals, run errands, fought with landlords, dealt with creditors, walked dogs, helped with laundry, changed light bulbs, shoveled snow, and picked up items from the store or pharmacy.

Several years ago, in Florida, a lovely elderly gentleman was referred to our agency for health-related issues. During the admission process, he patiently answered my questions, signed forms, and allowed me to complete the required nursing assessment. When I got to the questions related to sleep, he described an unusual scenario of a long series of sleepless nights.

"Every night when I try to sleep and the apartment is quiet," Mr. Bennett said, "a cricket wakes me up. I've had this crazy cricket for weeks, and I'm just about at my wit's end."

"Really?" I replied, not quite sure where to go with that.

"My buddy is going to pick me up some traps today. I'll get that cricket if it's the last thing I do!"

"Well, good for you," I said as I gathered my things to go. "I hope you catch it."

At the next visit, I was curious to hear how the cricket traps had worked out.

"No dice!" he said with disgust. "I'm starting to think it might not be crickets. Did you know that palmetto bugs make a noise too?"

I'd learned that a person can't live in Florida without having some up close and personal experiences with palmetto bugs. These large, winged cousins of the common cockroach give most people the willies, and believe me, I was no exception. However, to my knowledge they never made a peep, and I said as much as I checked his blood pressure and made notations in his chart.

"Don't be too sure," he said at last. "It's a more shrill noise than crickets make, and I'm pretty certain that's what it is. I have to catch it if I'm ever going to get a good night's sleep."

And so the quest for the palmetto bug continued.

Each visit, as I addressed his health issues, Mr. Bennett regaled me with his latest attempts to catch his nemesis. This went on for several weeks, until one day during our visit he suddenly paused and held up his hand.

"There!" he said excitedly. "Did you hear it? Now that crazy bug is starting in during the daytime! When will it ever end?"

"Are you talking about that faint chirp?" I asked him with a smile.

"Yeah it sounds faint now, but not in the middle of the night, believe me," he said with exasperation.

I heard it again, and this time, I was sure.

"Mr. Bennett," I said, "would you mind if I stood on your kitchen chair for a minute?"

Puzzled, he shook his head and gave me the go-ahead.

Carrying the chair back into the hallway, I set it down, stepped up, opened the smoke detector, and removed the batteries. The alarm gave one final chirp.

"You don't have a cricket or a palmetto bug," I said, as I showed him the spent batteries. "All you need is some new batteries."

"That's what's been keeping me up all night?" he asked with disbelief. "Not a bug after all?"

"That's it," I said with a smile. "The only thing that's been bugging you is this smoke detector."

He shook his head in disbelief. "All this time, and it was as simple as that."

"If you have some new batteries," I said, "I'll be happy to change them for you."

He produced the new batteries, which I inserted with a flourish, snapping the lid back in place.

"There you go," I said as I carried the chair back to his kitchen table, and mentally added this task to my unusual-things-I-have-done-in-the-course-of-work list.

"Honey" he said, "that was worth a million dollars to me."

Smiling, I patted his shoulder and then gathered my things to go. "I can't wait to hear about how well you slept the next time I come back."

"And I can't wait to sleep!" he exclaimed.

Mr. Bennett greeted me with a wide smile at our next and final visit.

"I'm a new man!" he said as he opened the door. "Best sleep I've had in weeks!"

~Sharon Stoika-Smay

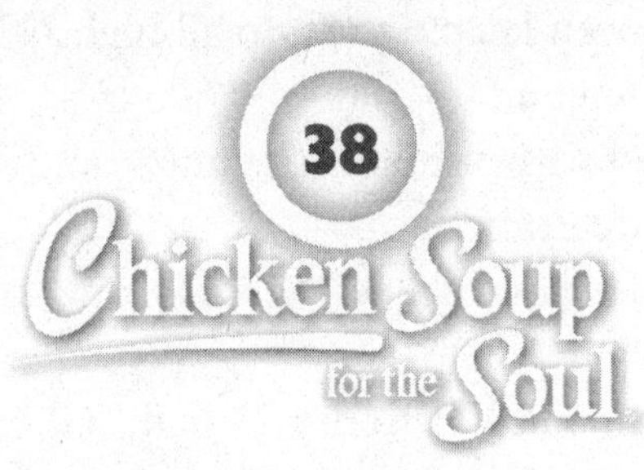

Nurse Jesse

It is not how much we do — it is how much love we put into the doing.
~Mother Teresa

The room was dark save for the green glow of monitors, yet I sensed his presence before I opened my eyes, made heavy by morphine. He stood with his back to me. I watched as he replaced the IV bag suspended from a pole.

He turned. "So, you're awake."

"Who're you?" I asked.

So many doctors, nurses and technicians had been in and out of my hospital room that I once mistook a uniformed maintenance man for a member of the medical team. I had blurted out my bowel concerns before he had a chance to tell me he was there to fix the radiator.

The man flipped a switch on a monitor and took a step closer to my bed. "I'm Jesse," he said. "Your nurse. There was a shift change while you were sleeping. Becky's gone for the night."

"Oh," I said, taking in this new information. More changes. "I need the bathroom."

"Okay. Just a minute. Shade your eyes." Jesse flipped on the overhead light.

He had brown skin, shiny black hair, and light blue scrubs like a surgeon. He was my first male nurse and didn't fit the old picture stuck in my head. When I was a kid, nurses were mostly perky young women in white caps and dresses.

Jesse helped me sit up. The thick gauze turban swaddling my head made me feel top heavy, and the drugs made me woozy. I counted three IV lines attached to ports inserted into my arm. Jesse maneuvered the IV pole so I wouldn't get tangled. He placed a walker in front of me. I didn't think I could stand and I told him so.

"You can do it," he said. I stretched my toes to the floor and shifted my weight onto one foot and then the other, gripping the walker. Jesse wheeled the IV pole along beside me, put a firm hand on the small of my back, and guided me the few steps to the bathroom.

"I'll be right here," he said, as he closed the door.

After I was back in bed, Jesse asked me if I had been able to urinate. I nodded.

"Okay, let's see how you did."

Jesse pushed a cart up next to the bed and explained the ultrasound machine he'd use to measure the volume of liquid remaining in my bladder. He rolled the wand back and forth on my lower abdomen and frowned. "Your bladder is still pretty full. If you can't empty it you'll need a catheter."

"No!" I cried out in a panic. "Not that!" It had been almost two months since I was diagnosed with a brain tumor. Thank God it was benign. I was through with being a patient. I didn't want any tubes tying me to that hospital bed. I wanted to go home.

"What's wrong?" Jesse asked softly. "It would just be temporary."

I couldn't answer as I choked back tears.

Jesse pulled a chair up next to my bed and sat down. I eyed him with curiosity, wondering just how long he would wait for my answer. I had become accustomed to the fast-pace of the hospital staff, which allowed no time for conversation. I was in a teaching hospital, and when a doctor with a group of med students crowded around my bed, I felt like a lab rat under observation. Questions to me were focused on the physical: On a scale of one to ten, what's your pain level? How's your appetite? Are you drinking? Have you gone to the bathroom yet? No one had seemed interested in what was going on in my heart or mind.

Jesse leaned back in the chair and rested his arms in his lap.

"I'm afraid of a catheter," I said. "Before my dad died he had a catheter and he hated it. I felt so bad for him. Catheters remind me how much he suffered. And how I couldn't help him. I just don't want one."

Jesse paused a moment. "Okay. Then let's see what we can do. You rest for a little while longer, then I'll get you up again and we'll walk the hall. Walking usually helps."

Jesse sat with me. We talked. He asked about my work and my family and about what I liked to do. He didn't ask about my brain tumor. He talked to me like a friend, not a patient. Though his primary responsibility was with my body, he was as interested in what concerned me and what brought me joy. For the first time in a long time, I felt like more than a wrecked car in a body shop.

When I was rested, Jesse helped me stand up again and I wrapped my fingers around the IV pole. He took hold of my other arm. Each step was an effort, but he supported me and we walked partway down the hall and back. It was exhausting. When we returned to the room, he steered me into the bathroom.

After I was back in bed, he ran the wand over my bladder again.

"Better," he said. "But not good enough. You're not empty."

I groaned, expecting him to bring up the catheter again. But no, Jesse sat back down in the chair and I relaxed back into the pillows.

It took two more strolls, separated by dozing and conversation, before he repeated the ultrasound and proclaimed, "Empty!"

All night I'd felt as though I were Jesse's only patient, though I knew that he had others. When he finally left my room, dawn was breaking. I fell back to sleep feeling abundantly grateful. I had been cared for in body, heart and mind.

~Lorri Danzig

Unresponsive

When we accept tough jobs as a challenge and wade into them with joy and enthusiasm, miracles can happen.
~Harry S. Truman

After a few days off, I came back to work at the extended care unit and heard report on my patients. One young woman, a new patient, stood out.

The night nurse said. "She had a severe brain injury and is unable to speak or understand. She's unresponsive, incurable. She has a retention catheter and has to be fed."

I got her breakfast tray, and as was my custom with new patients, responsive or not, I began to talk to her. "Good morning, my name is Irene," I said. "I will be your nurse for the next few days. I am going to feed you your breakfast now."

As I fed this young pretty woman, I continued talking as if she could understand me.

Suddenly she spoke. "Every time I open my mouth you put something in it."

I stood up, stunned, staring at her as she repeated it. I put down the fork. "Excuse me for a minute. I'll be right back." I raced to the head nurse and told her what had just happened.

"What?" she said. "That isn't possible. Her records say and her husband confirmed that she can't talk or understand because of the severe brain injury."

"Well," I said, "she can talk!" I went back to finish feeding her, and as I talked to her, she spoke. This "unresponsive" woman was speaking and understanding!

All the nurses were excited and dedicated to her recovery now. We made a plan to speed her progress. When any of us entered the room we would talk to her and not leave until she answered, no matter what. If we said, "Good morning," she had to reply, "Good morning." If we asked her how she was, she had to answer with something.

Within a couple of weeks we didn't have to wait long and she began talking before we did. Her husband was astounded. He coaxed her to respond to him, too.

It didn't take long before she was feeding herself, combing her own hair and sitting up on her own. However, she still had to be in a wheelchair and needed assistance from the bed to the chair.

One day, she asked, "Can you take this catheter out?" She was worried about wetting the bed but she wanted to try living without the catheter. The nursing staff promised that we would come ASAP to assist her to the bathroom as soon as she put her light on. The doctor agreed that she could try.

The first day the catheter was out, everyone on the floor, whether she was their patient or not, sprinted to her room like marathon runners whenever her bell light came on. It worked. She made it to the bathroom almost every time. After a while, she had better retention and we didn't need to race so fast.

Next, the goal was for her to walk. And she did, step by unsteady step, first with assistance, then eventually on her own.

Then one glorious day, this "unresponsive incurable" woman went home. Her loving husband, who thought he had lost his wife forever, extended his arm and she wove hers through his, and she walked out, to care for her young family and get on with her life.

~Gladys Swedak

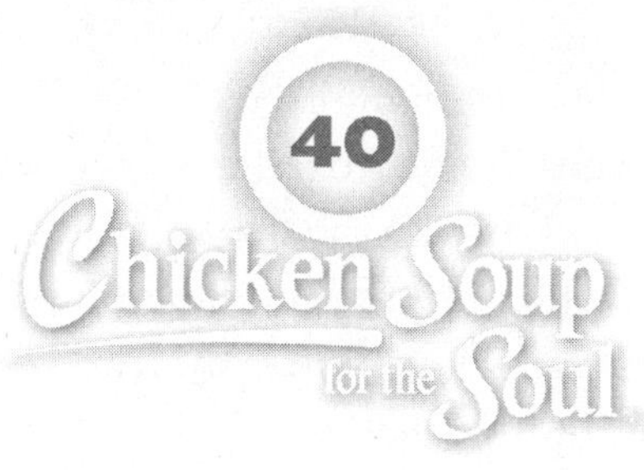

Float Pool: Sink or Swim

In helping others we shall help ourselves, for whatever good we give out completes the circle and comes back to us.
~Flora Edwards

"Why would nurses volunteer for Float Pool?" I wondered. It was like being a substitute teacher, having to be resourceful in so many areas. I was not fond of a changing work environment, so I admired these brave people.

One evening, during low census, I was drafted to fill Pool shortages. Hesitantly, I left my fifth floor dialysis unit and headed for seventh floor orthopedics, where I stopped cold. The charge nurse was buried in a disorganized pile of papers. The unit clerk's forehead flashed an invisible sign: "I dare you to speak to me." The day shift staff darted in and out of rooms to beat the clock. I wanted to bail out.

After some time, a disembodied voice asked if I was the float nurse. Instructed to "Wait," I stood around nearly twenty minutes holding my belongings. I already felt like I was sinking as I watched the commotion.

Frustrated, I took action and returned to the fifth floor, placed my dinner in the fridge, and printed out the Ortho census on that computer. I privately longed to stay, but returned to the seventh floor where the charge nurse had my assignment ready. She pointed me toward report.

I slid into the closest seat and took notes. There were no introductions; no one even acknowledged me. Hopelessly behind schedule, we all made a mad dash to the floor after report.

Back on the chaotic unit, I was trying to find a resource person when I heard a serious-looking nurse say, "Are you the float nurse?"

I was rescued! But my relief was short-lived. She wasn't there to help me; she wanted me to help her.

Through visible grief, the nurse begged me to spend my shift supporting Mrs. Smith, a terminally ill woman. I would have wholeheartedly done this had I not been given a heavy assignment on a busy disordered floor. She was handing me an anchor. The Ortho unit and equipment were unfamiliar to me. I had six people late for meds already and I didn't have an access code for medications. During report I'd learned that someone needed morphine ASAP. Someone else needed more IV fluids hung and the site was clotting. I was already drowning.

The nurse pleaded with me, but I knew Mrs. Smith deserved better than I could offer. I would be overextended and no one would receive good care. I gently explained I'd never met the dying woman and that she might feel more supported with a familiar nurse. With wide eyes and a new mission, the nurse ran off to change the assignment.

Still lacking resources, I returned to the fifth floor and used my code for meds. I also picked up supplies I couldn't access or find on the seventh floor. I'd straighten out logistics later. Back on Ortho, I saw Mrs. Smith's bed being pushed into a private room. I was relieved someone would meet her special needs.

My shift got no better. Nothing went smoothly; nothing was timely. Tasks were delayed while I sought information. I received a medication access code halfway through the shift. The previous nurse had let fluids run out so I had to restart IVs. I was behind schedule the entire shift and never did get that dinner I'd stored back on the fifth floor.

To make matters worse, working with unfamiliar orthopedic

equipment required hijacking another nurse to assist. I hated to bother anyone, but I had no choice. When I did track someone down, help was given cheerfully. I just didn't feel welcome to approach anyone since no one spoke to me.

My frustration paled next to the pity I felt for the patients expecting and deserving good nursing care. Being an unsupported float substitute robbed me of the opportunity to be the nurse I desired to be.

I staggered home after this awful experience, determined to effect change.

The next day I decided to write a thank-you note to the nurses on Ortho. Yes, a thank you note. Contradictory as it sounds, I had a plan.

Sending the note was easy. The hospital administration had recently implemented a system for relaying compliments and comments. Notecards displayed on suggestion boxes in each department read, "Let us know how we're doing." Visitors, clients, staff, and managers were encouraged to write comments, which were delivered directly to the hospital administrator. After adding a personal remark, she would forward the note to the appropriate department head, then to the manager or director of nursing, and finally to the employee.

I could have used this system to complain, but I knew it would be more productive to emphasize the positive. So I wrote about floating to Seven and being dependent on those nurses to share their Ortho knowledge. I named the people who had helped me, and thanked them. I complimented the compassionate nursing I'd observed. I named the nurse, a true advocate, who had been so concerned for the dying woman.

I knew their supervisors would acknowledge the nurses I praised. I hoped that would raise expectations. By saying the seventh floor nurses willingly helped floats, I set a precedent for all the nurses there, hopefully raising standards.

Next, I wanted to be sure floats had a positive experience on our unit. I told my coworkers about my dreadful shift and we agreed we didn't want that reputation for us. In fact, we wanted fifth floor dialysis to be the floats' favorite place to work.

From then on, we welcomed the float nurses right away and introduced ourselves, which generally surprised them. We created a buddy system, a place for personal belongings, and a designated communication slot for the floats. Assignments reflected the training and availability of the substitute. We treated that nurse like a guest and checked in often. Immediately following the shift, we all signed a compliment card, thanking him or her for working with us.

The results amazed us. With VIP treatment for our floats, the atmosphere felt like a holiday. All staff members were happier and less stressed. I'm sure this led to better patient care.

We received thank you cards from the floats for making them feel supported. Our staff received compliment notes from hospital and nursing administrators stating their appreciation of our special efforts to improve the work environment. Patients and visitors sent us cheerful compliment cards.

As an unexpected benefit, our Keep-the-Float-Afloat plan spread to other units. When one of our nurses floated, she returned with news of being treated very well, even on Seven. When Five and Seven became favorite places to float, I knew my plan had worked.

As we suspected, a supported float nurse rises to the top and everyone swims — I mean, wins.

~Elizabeth Rae

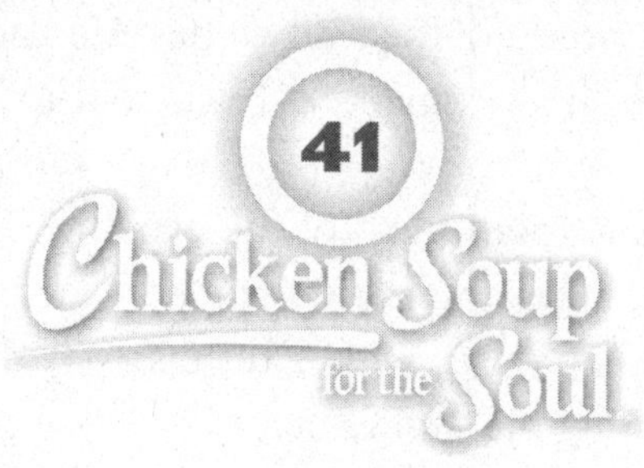

Inappropriate

The most wasted of all days is one without laughter.
~E. E. Cummings

I had come from working a year on night shift at the pediatric unit to second shift on the mental health wing. Needless to say, I had a huge learning curve.

I loved it from the first day, when Lester swung his invisible sword over my left shoulder to protect me from an invisible dragon attack. He was one of the sweetest men I'd met. But as I quickly found out, many of the men were not as kind.

When mental illness, medication reactions, or withdrawal affect a person, incredibly shocking and unsavory things often get flung the nurse's way. And with me being the youngest on staff and infuriatingly prone to blushing, I became a really easy target.

At my six-month evaluation, my manager encouraged me greatly by saying I "belonged" as a psych nurse. To be counted among the best, and weirdest, nurses I'd known was an honor.

But when it came to discussing obstacles, I admitted my biggest was handling sexual or inappropriate comments from male patients. So she made one of my yearly goals to be "more self-assertive and upfront in setting appropriate verbal boundaries with patients and advocating respect" for myself.

So, fresh with new empowerment, I walked to the nurse's station for report to find I was assigned a disgruntled and unhappy man who had been very rude to the staff all day. He had a heavy lisp and supposedly did not like women, so I was told to be firm and listen carefully.

He stayed in his room most of the evening. The shift had been calm and we were all gathering our nightly meds when I saw him charging around the corner with a deep frown, furrowed forehead and a blanket draping his shoulders.

He stopped just short of the door and put both hands on his hips. His eyes locked on mine as he angrily blurted, "Can we have sex tonight?"

I thought, "Deep breath, here's your chance. Calm the blush down."

"Sir, that is highly inappropriate and you cannot speak to me that way," I said with my best faux-confidence.

His face twisted with anger and his voice got louder as he shouted incredulously, "But we had sex *last* night!"

I squared my shoulders, set my jaw. "We most certainly did not! I'm going to have to insist you speak to me in a respectful way. You are being very inappropriate."

The vein in his forehead started to throb and I thought I'd have to call security, he was so livid.

"Fine by me," I thought with some pride. I had stood up for myself.

He threw up his hands and shouted so loud I jumped, "What in the world is inappropriate about popcorn?"

I stopped mentally patting my back long enough to ask, "Wait, you said 'sex' right?"

"No!" he bellowed. "Shnacks!"

Oooh. The lisp. The evening movie night. Accompanied by the evening popcorn.

All that earlier empowerment disappeared as the cackles of my fellow nurses dissolved into fits of uncontrollable laughter. My face darkened five shades and I sputtered, "Sir, I'm… I'm so sorry… I thought you were asking for sex… not snacks."

He stood up straight, took the dragging corner of his hospital blanket and whipped it around his shoulder like an indignant Zorro as he raised his hand and pointed at me. "Now that, young lady, is inappropriate."

Then he stormed off, Orville Redenbacher in hand.

~Cassidy Doolittle

The Champ

What does it take to be a champion? Desire, dedication, determination, concentration and the will to win.
~Patty Berg

Tim was a fifth grader when I met him. He had autism and some physical challenges, one of which was severe congenital anatomical problems that made it impossible for him to control his bowels. He wore adult diapers and had a regimented daily bowel program. Odor was always a problem, which as he became older became a social issue too.

Tim and I bonded immediately. He was a funny young man, obsessed with professional wrestling. So, being a non-athlete myself, I asked my college-age son, Larry, to give me a quick lesson on World Wrestling Entertainment and John Cena, Tim's favorite wrestler. I learned enough to equal a fifth grader's knowledge, and Larry gave me daily updates on John Cena's record, matches, personality traits and the world of WWE.

I saw Tim every day because he used my health office bathroom for his bowel program and his adult diaper needs. We had to have many talks about his hygiene and the odor issue when he did not change frequently enough. We always talked about Mr. Cena, who Tim referred to only as "The Champ."

One day, when Tim was in seventh grade, he was in my freshly painted bathroom late in the day and I heard him using the room deodorizer spray. When I came in the next morning, I gasped to see CHAMP, THE CHAMP, WWE, and JOHN CENA written all over the walls. Tim claimed he didn't know the room deodorizer would stain the walls. I, of course, had to report it and Tim, of course, had to help repaint the bathroom.

Tim's grandmother did a fabulous job raising Tim and his siblings. We spoke often and she knew I would do whatever I could to help. We talked a lot about his bowel issues. So far he had not been teased about it, but I was sure that was on the horizon. Hopefully girls were on the horizon too. It took many conversations and much convincing for her to see that he was a young man facing social stigmas and if surgical corrections could be made, this was the time to do it. It still took several years before Grandmom took him to a surgeon, but surgery was eventually scheduled.

I left the middle school for a high school job. Tim, Grandmom, and I lost touch.

Several years passed and on one of the worst days of my life, the day of my mother's funeral, my phone rang. My home was filled with company when my husband called me to the phone, not recognizing the name of Tim's grandmother on the caller ID. It seems that they thought about me as much as I thought about them. She wanted me to know that Tim had his surgery and how it had changed their lives. He went on to high school and was thriving beautifully with friends. We chatted for a while and I thanked her for making that awful day brighter.

Several years later, I was in the waiting room of one of my physicians when in walked Tim and his grandmother! He was all grown up, tall and thin, but still had that quality about him I will never forget. His voice had deepened and he had a scruffy beard but we recognized each other immediately.

"CHAMP!" he shouted. He eagerly told me he was in community college studying computer software and he was close to earning his degree. He had a colostomy that he cared for himself, a girlfriend, and he still loved WWE and THE CHAMP. With the help of medication, he had overcome many of his learning difficulties and was doing better than he ever thought possible.

The tears in my eyes clouded the light in his.

~Lynn B. Zoll

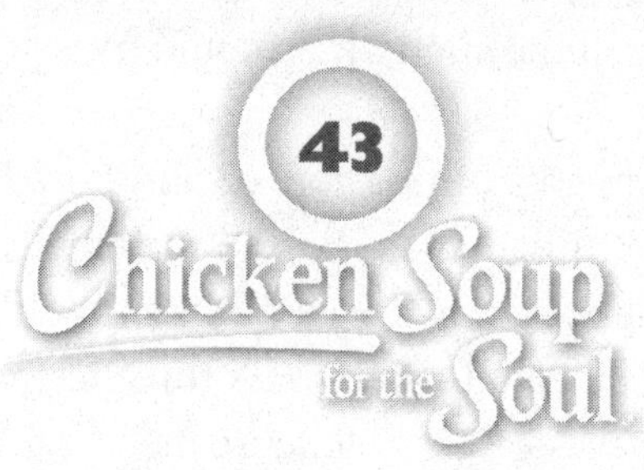

Coping

He didn't tell me how to live; he lived, and let me watch him do it.
~Clarence Budington Kelland

My father's bed was at the foot of my own. I would lie there and listen as his breaths became longer and shallower. I held my breath as I waited for him to take his next.

I'd taken a leave of absence from work to be his primarily caregiver, along with my brother and mom. Dad's esophageal cancer had metastasized throughout his entire body and we vowed to make him comfortable with home hospice care.

Eventually I had to go back to work after my leave. Within the first hour I was back on the job, my dad passed away. Mom and Grandmother told me he had used his last bit of strength to hold on, so as not to die in front of me.

Caring for Dad changed me forever. I decided to become a registered nurse.

Years later, at the start of my shift, I walked into a patient's room to introduce myself, as I always do. Mr. Jones was in his late sixties, sick with cancer and admitted due to shortness of breath.

Just like Dad.

When I asked how he was doing he said, "Just fine," though he was obviously in discomfort and his respirations labored. Between each breath, he answered my questions with a smile on his face, which looked as if it took all the strength he could muster.

Just like Dad.

After a few moments of our conversation, all I could see was my dad when Mom and I had taken him to the emergency room because of his extreme pain. Dad had joked with the admitting nurse and laughed, although he could barely walk three feet without gasping.

Now Mr. Jones was gasping. "Excuse me," I said. "I'll be back soon, but first I want to check on your medications."

But what I really meant was that I had to find a quiet place to hide and try not to cry.

Since my father's passing, I hadn't been in a situation that had brought on the same emotions I'd had caring for him. Being the manly man that I was, I couldn't let people see me near tears. I wanted to take a long break. Or switch patients. But I didn't do either.

I found an unoccupied room, took deep breaths, and wiped my eyes. I couldn't allow my emotions to stop me from caring for a patient in need. I thought back to my dad's laughter during his last days and how strong he was, never uttering one word of complaint. Visualizing his smile, his positivity, and his strength fortified mine. I thought of all those nurses at the hospital and hospice who had cared for my dad and family, and I tapped into their strength.

I took a few more deep breaths, squared my shoulders, and reentered Mr. Jones's room. I gave him the best care possible that day, and the next… and the next.

A few months after he was discharged, my nursing unit received a card from him and his family saying how they appreciated the care given him. And his cancer was in remission!

As I read the card, I recalled the day when my own tumult had interrupted his care, and was reminded again how we nurses often have to help patients and families cope with difficult situations and emotions while finding ways to cope with our own.

In those situations I continue to perform my duties and care for my patients with a smile on my face, with all the strength I can muster.

Just like Dad.

~Alioune Kotey

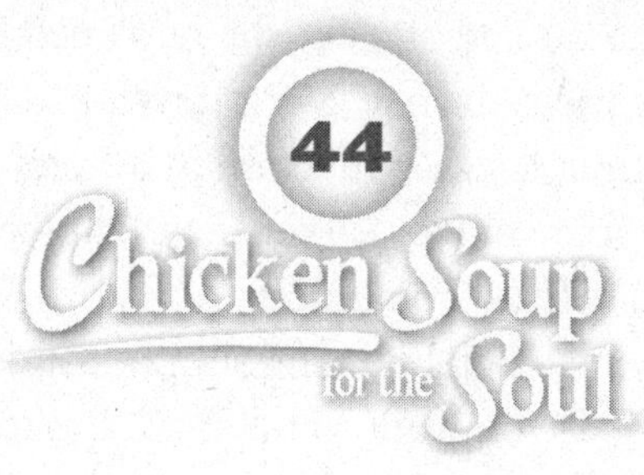

Three Elephants

When old people speak it is not because of the sweetness of words in our mouths; it is because we see something which you do not see.

~Chinua Achebe

On my final visit, Mary was feeling bad. I could tell as soon as I walked in. She was seated in her wheelchair and her face was pale with pain, her eyes rheumy.

Her daughter Winnie met me at the door. "Mother has something to tell you," she said, knotting her hands together anxiously.

My heart thrummed like hummingbird wings. I had no idea what Mary had to say, but I was worried.

Although I had been a nurse for twenty-five years, I was still new to home health. On average, I drove 800 miles a week through three large, rural counties. It meant very long days, often with unexpected situations in patients' homes.

I had met Mary and her husband Herbert almost a year before. A spry octogenarian couple from the great Northwest, they had ventured to the deserts of the arid Southwest to visit Winnie. During the vacation, Mary took a tumble, fracturing her right arm and shoulder. My visits had included many hours of excruciating exercises and loving conversations. I was closer to Mary than any patient I'd ever cared for.

They stayed at Winnie's, and over time Mary's fractures healed and her pain became more tolerable, but she remained limited to a wheelchair. Then to our great dismay, Mary developed bowel cancer. She didn't have much time left. My function as a home health nurse suddenly shifted to hospice nurse. Rather than help her body heal, I was doing all I could to help as it shut down.

I put down my big bag of nursing supplies and went over to pale, stoic Mary. "What is it you want to tell me?" I asked, kneeling beside her.

"Give me your hand," she said solemnly.

I extended my hand, palm open. I tried not shake, having no idea what to expect. I could swear I saw tears in her eyes.

Mary smiled warmly and took my hand in her swollen hands. "I am going to tell you a story about three elephants." She started tracing little circles in the palm of my hand with her knobby index finger.

"Once there were three elephants: a great big papa elephant, a great big mama elephant, and a small baby elephant." She continued making circles in my palm.

"They were walking and walking in the jungle until Papa Elephant roared with his trunk and said, 'I need to go.' And he went over here." She moved her finger down to the tip of my thumb. "They kept walking and walking in the jungle and Mama Elephant trumpeted with her trunk and said, 'I need to go.' And she went over here." She moved her finger along my middle finger.

"They continued walking and walking through the jungle and Baby Elephant gave a toot with his trunk and said, 'I need to go.' And he went over here." Just as her finger drew a line to my pinkie, warm moisture dripped over my palm.

I jerked my hand away and stared at it. The baby elephant had just urinated on my hand!

Mary, Herbert, and Winnie roared with laughter. Mary mischievously opened her fist and revealed a water-soaked tissue.

For a minute I could only gawk. After all, Mary was dying. This was no time for a joke! But then I watched the pain melt away from her body as it shook with giggles. Then laughter bubbled out of all of us.

The next week, Mary was gone. Her family invited me to join in celebrating her life. Together, Herbert, Winnie, and I recounted all the wonderful times Mary had shared with us. We circled her life, like elephants walking around the jungle, laughing as much as we could along the way.

Today, I try to bring a bit of Mary's laughter to the hands I hold and the lives I touch.

~Donna Mason

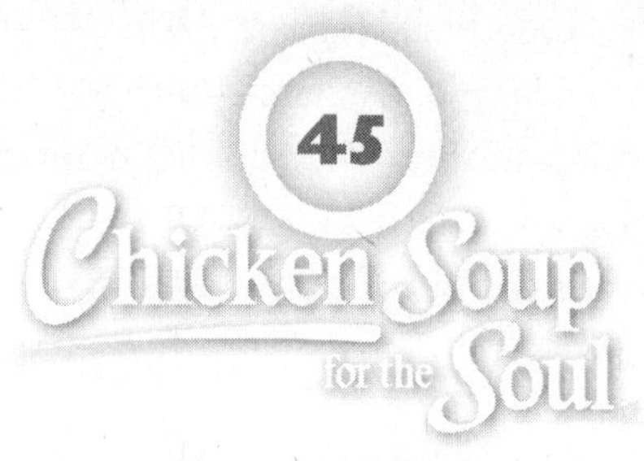

In the Sweet By and By

Music is well said to be the speech of angels.
~Thomas Carlyle

My brother asked me to come to the hospital one evening. The matriarch from my childhood church was not doing well and the family was requesting support.

When I arrived I could hear her heavy labored breathing from the hallway. The family was not sure what to do as they watched their beloved mother/grandmother struggle for breath. She had changed her status to Do Not Resuscitate, and they wanted to keep her comfortable. But she didn't look comfortable. As a hospice nurse I knew medications could make a difference and asked their permission to discuss changes to her plan of care with the nurse.

Unfortunately, it was not easy to make changes. It was the first week of the new electronic medical record and the computers were slow and the doctor didn't answer our phone call.

Knowing how important her faith had been all her life and how helpless the family and I felt while waiting to get orders, I suggested we sing some hymns. We closed the door so we wouldn't bother the patients in the neighboring rooms and started to sing.

We sang "What a Day That Will Be," "Because He Lives," "When

We All Get to Heaven," and finally, "In the Sweet By and By." As we finished that fourth hymn, she grew quiet. No more struggling to breathe. She had peacefully left her old worn-out body.

I opened the door to tell her nurse and was surprised to find all the staff from the floor standing right outside. "She passed," I said.

"We know. We saw it on the monitor. It was so beautiful we didn't want to interrupt."

It *was* beautiful. We had sung her to heaven.

~Kathy Stringham

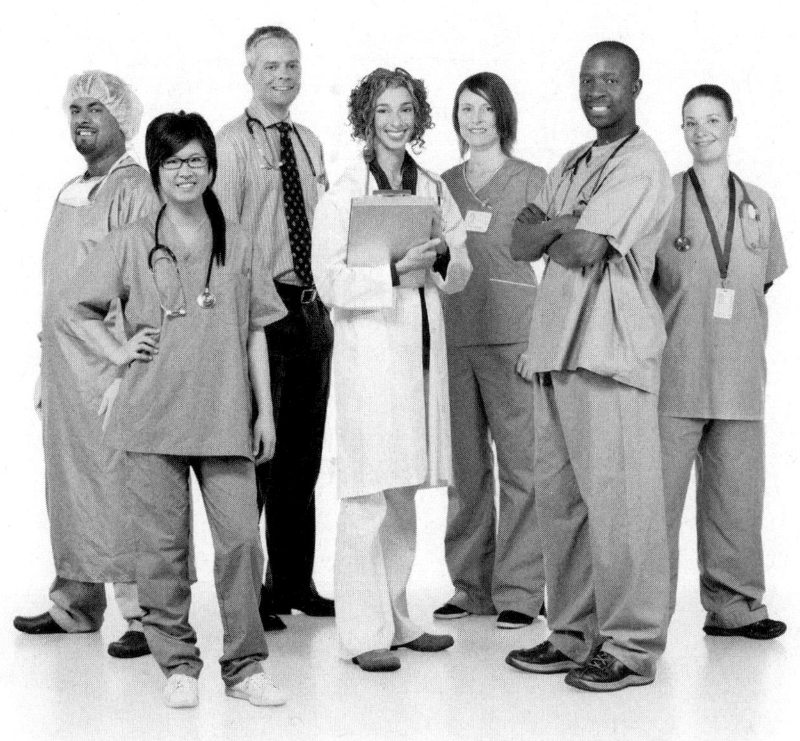

Inspiration for Nurses

Divine Intervention

A miracle is a work exceeding the power of any created agent, consequently being an effect of the divine omnipotence.

~Robert South

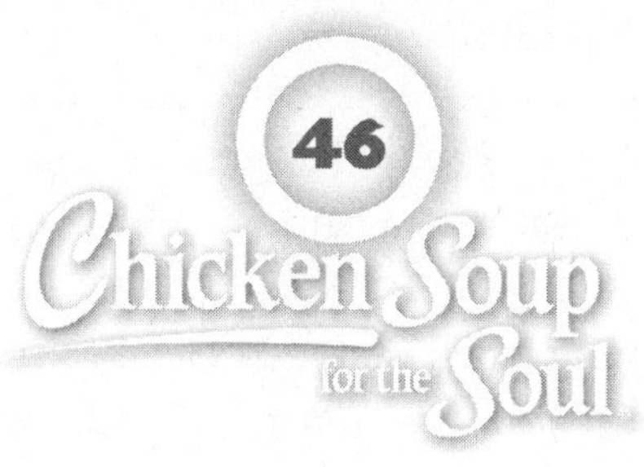

Hope for the Hurting

Very truly I tell you, whoever believes in me will do the works I have been doing, and they will do even greater things than these.
~John 14:12 NIV

It can be very frustrating caring for someone in uncontrollable pain. You feel helpless sometimes, especially when there is no cure. You treat the symptoms and wish to God you could give them more. So you listen, without rushing them, offering a hand to gently hold, looking into their eyes and letting them know they are not alone, that there is hope.

I tried to keep Dianne as comfortable as possible within my scope of practice. Pain meds, massage, heating pad, pillows. Why was this happening to her? So young. So sad. Her stage IV cancer had metastasized throughout her spine and she was in severe and almost constant pain.

Every three hours I went into her room and medicated her. I asked her what felt better as I tried to gently position her; sometimes just a tiny movement of a pillow brought a little relief.

When my shift was ending I went to Dianne's room to say goodnight. I told her I would see her again in the morning. "I will keep you in my prayers," I said. She nodded her head and looked out her window.

I drove home, took a quick shower, got dressed and drove to my friend Sue's house for dinner.

After dinner we prayed together. I remembered Dianne and I sincerely prayed, "Lord, I pray that you will run your fingers along Dianne's spine and heal her of cancer," while visualizing that in my mind.

The next morning when I entered Dianne's room she was beaming like a child on Christmas morning. "Did you go to church last night?"

"No, I didn't go to church, but I did go to my friend's house and we had a prayer meeting."

Dianne beamed a big effervescent smile, her eyebrows lifted in excitement, her countenance filled with joy. "Did you remember to pray for me?"

"Yes, as a matter of fact we had special prayer for you."

"I felt you praying for me! So I started praying too. It was around nine o'clock, right?"

I nodded.

"This sounds crazy, but I felt God touch me. Really! And all the pain left. I haven't taken any pain medications since!"

Indeed, the doctor taking care of her was astounded; he had no explanation for what happened. He ordered more tests. Dianne's cancer was completely gone.

I've learned that while caring for my patients, I include the Great Physician in partnership with me. He gives hope to the hopeless. As nurses we are but instruments in the hand of the One who heals, and we can expect miracles.

~Elizabeth Carroll

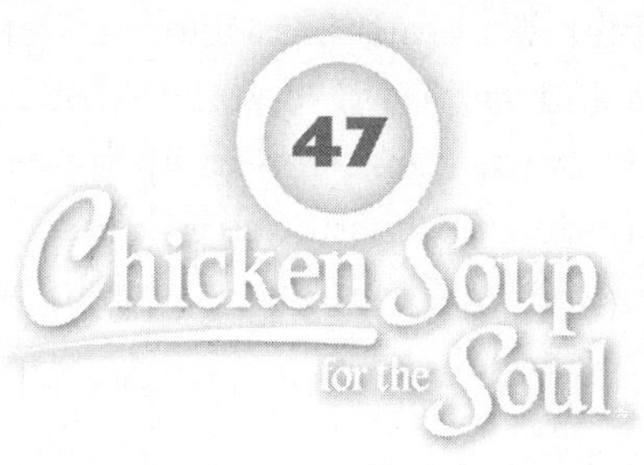

Bernadette

The bonds of love are what connect us to the other side.
~John Edward

Bernadette was eighty-four years young and too weak to walk on her own. Three of her best friends wheeled her into her hospice room and promptly informed me that she liked her martinis, cigarettes and dancing.

Bernadette had a gleam in her eye and a joke on her tongue each morning as I assessed her. She was feisty, funny… and a bit afraid. She often asked, "Am I dying?"

I answered, "Only God knows."

Between our serious conversations, she made me laugh.

One day Bernadette grew much weaker. She gestured toward the window and said, "Do you see Susie?"

I looked where she pointed.

Bernadette had a dreamy look on her face and her eyes stared in wonder. "Susie is there and she's so beautiful."

I carried on with my busy day while Bernadette mostly slept. Around dinnertime her daughter-in-law Mary arrived. "How's Bernadette doing today?"

I informed her that Bernadette was indeed declining, then said, "She saw a beautiful girl named Susie this morning."

Mary was amazed. She jumped back and leaned against the wall. She finally said, "Seventy-eight years ago, Bernadette lost her six-year-old daughter in a drowning accident. Her name was Susie."

I was shocked and saddened to realize that this feisty, fun, martini-loving lady had borne the sorrow of losing her only daughter for many years. No wonder she'd had such a look of wonder on her face. She beheld her beautiful little girl who came to take her in her arms to spend eternity together.

~Christine Bielecki

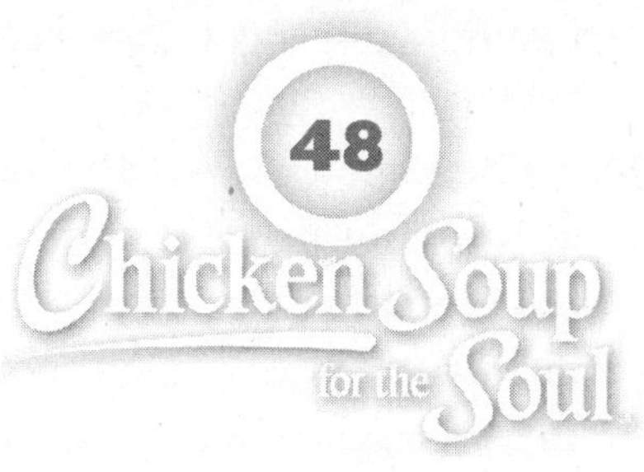

I'm Going Home

Duty is ours, results are God's.
~John Quincy Adams

I was a new nurse and for a week had been caring for an eighty-year-old highly decorated World War II hero who had flown many daring missions. But now he was confused, disoriented to time and place. He often spoke of his urgent need to get to his next mission, or he'd wake suddenly, terrified he'd be late for bugle call. I soothed him and he'd calm down for a while. His health was failing rapidly and he was too weak to walk, so we lifted him into a chair twice daily, which seemed to make him happy.

His wife of sixty years brought pictures of him in his uniform. I could, with a little imagination, see the remains of a dashing young man in his old ravaged body. She wanted us to see all he was and had been. She was also elderly and in poor health, and it was with great difficulty that she came to visit him every day. She kissed him on arrival each morning, and his eyes lit up. She held his hand or stroked his brow as he drifted in and out of sleep, comforted by her presence.

One day he attempted to get out of bed by himself, saying, "It is finally time for me to go!"

I rushed to his side to keep him from falling." You don't have to go right now. Why don't you rest a while first?"

He calmed briefly, then insisted, "I need to go right away, it's time!"

I was amazed at the change in him. He seemed stronger, and

his vital signs were more stable than they had been since his hospitalization.

His wife called to let him know she would visit a little later than usual. He told her, with great urgency, "I really need to go! You have to hurry and get here so I can leave!"

Remembering that distraction is a good tool in dealing with dementia, I put him in a wheelchair and placed him by the nurse's station where he smiled and nodded to everyone who passed.

An hour later he called down the hall to me: "Brenda." I was surprised and pleased that he recognized me. I took his hands in mine.

"I don't have much time left," he said. "I need to go."

"Do you want to go back to bed?"

He smiled but shook his head. "No," he said patiently. "I just need to go home."

As a dutiful new nurse, I explained, "I ordered you a great lunch, and your wife will be here soon to feed you. How about waiting until after lunch to go?"

He nodded reluctantly, but agreed. Just then his wife arrived. She was overjoyed to see him out of his room. He laughed when he saw her, and called to her. His lunch tray was waiting, so we took him back to his room. He shook my hand, then pulled me to him and hugged me. "Thank you for taking such good care of me, Brenda."

I was speechless, overcome with tears and emotion. I hugged him back. "It's my privilege, Mr. Smith, my honor."

After lunch, I returned to his room. His wife stood beside his bed, an odd look on her face. "He kept telling me all morning he needed to leave, that it was his time to go. He was so excited."

"He told me the same thing," I said, looking fondly at him as he slept.

"Oh, Brenda," she said in a gentle voice. "I think he's gone."

I looked at her in disbelief, then back at him. I placed my fingers on his radial pulse and my stethoscope over his heart. My eyes blurred with tears. It was true.

"But, I don't understand! He was doing so well!" I blurted.

"He was trying to tell us that he was ready to die, but we didn't realize it."

I put my arms around her, and we both began to cry.

She said, "I will never forget what you did for us."

When I called the doctor, I conveyed the morning's events. "But I don't understand the sudden change."

The wise old physician told me something I have never forgotten. "Sometimes God, in His infinite wisdom, allows a dying person a really good day just before he dies. And sometimes God, in His infinite love, allows that patient's family the comfort of seeing their loved one experience that good day. And sometimes God, in His infinite grace, allows us to be a part of it."

~Brenda Stiverson

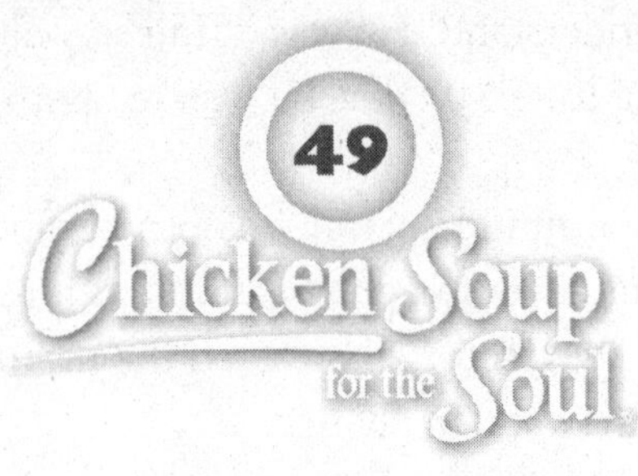

Nothing Is Impossible

The miracles on earth are the laws of heaven.
~Jean Paul

Mr. J was admitted to our hospital unresponsive. His CT scan showed a huge inter-cranial hemorrhage and he was rushed to surgery to relieve the pressure. His recovery was very slow in the Surgical Intensive Care Unit. Eventually he became stable enough to be transferred to the Progressive Care and Stroke Unit.

A Hispanic man in his sixties, Mr. J had a stroke twenty years prior to this admission, leaving him with right-sided hemiparesis. Amazingly, he went back to school after his stroke and became a high school teacher.

Mr. J had been in the hospital for three months by this time and was unresponsive except for opening his eyes. He was also non-verbal except for moaning sounds. I took care of him many times and each time his baseline remained unchanged.

It was a Saturday morning when I walked in to see how he was doing. He looked the same as every other time I'd assessed him. Except maybe, just maybe, I saw a twinge of movement in his right hand. I dismissed it as wishful thinking. Besides, it was pretty minimal, if it was anything at all, so I began rounding with my other patients, doing assessments, giving meds, reviewing the labs, and calling doctors for orders—the normal routine.

Over the years I have learned that sometimes God enters our "normal" and brings a "supernatural" manifestation that even doctors cannot explain. As I give care to my patients, I try to be alert for the supernatural. I strive to give excellent care as a nurse, and also keep the window open for the miraculous. I have seen it too many times to not believe.

Sunday morning on my way to the hospital, I prayed for my patients to be healed, as I did most mornings. After I got report from the night nurse, I walked into Mr. J's room and said, "Good morning." He looked the same, and his assessment was unchanged, so I went back to the desk to chart. I noticed the night nurse had also charted that his right side was flaccid, no movement.

I started feeling a little annoyed. Had I seen a tiny bit of movement the day before or not? I got up from the desk and walked back into his room and did something I had never done in my nursing career. I didn't ask him if he could move, I commanded him. "Lift up your right leg." He lifted his right leg off the bed! A leg that hadn't moved for twenty years!

He looked at me in awe. "Am I doing that?" I had never heard him talk before.

"Yes! You are doing it!"

Excitedly, I said, "Lift your right arm." And sure enough he did!

Next came his hand, and he grasped mine.

I ran to the front desk and called the house supervisor and then phoned the patient's neurosurgeon. "I know we always call you to give you bad news and I want you to know that your patient who was paralyzed for twenty years can now lift his leg and keep it up in the air. And he speaks!"

I called Mr. J's daughter and asked her to come in to see her dad. When she got there, I took her in to see her father. Mr. J. was smiling like a child who had a secret. When we had her full attention, he lifted up his right arm and then his leg.

She started weeping. "This is a miracle!" Throwing her arms around her dad, with tears flowing down her cheeks, she pulled out her cell phone and began calling her family. "Dad's no longer paralyzed!"

During my shift, Mr. J. kept pushing his call light, something he had never done in the months he had been there. When I went into his room to see what he needed, he told me that an alarm was going off in the next room. He was right! Mr. J. was so alert, he was looking out for the patient in the next room. Even the cognitive part of his brain was back.

We nurses all know it's impossible for atrophied muscles, unused for twenty years, to work again. But we also know, nothing is impossible with God.

~Elizabeth Carroll

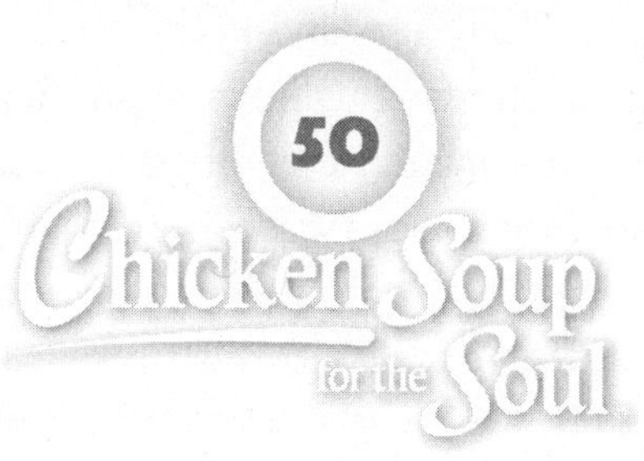

A Nurse's Christmas Prayer

Prayer is aligning ourselves with the purposes of God.
~E. Stanley Jones

On an early December morning in my home in Australia, I was startled awake by the phone ringing at my bedside. On the screen I saw the name of the nursing home where my father resided with Alzheimer's disease. I jerked upright and my heart pounded. I knew something was wrong. A voice gently but professionally said, "I'm so sorry. Your father had a massive stroke about ten minutes ago. He's had three seizures and is unconscious." She advised me to contact my mum and the family to go there as soon as possible.

We met at the nursing home with hugs and tears. We were grateful Dad was still alive, even if just long enough for us to say goodbye.

His doctor phoned us and said, "I have instructed the sister to give your father morphine to keep him comfortable. There is nothing else to do."

I asked, "So he can't make it back from this? Are you saying just keep him medicated until he passes away?"

The doctor replied, "Yes."

The kind nursing staff brought in extra chairs for us, plus trays of tea, coffee, sandwiches and biscuits, even drinks for the children. The compassion on the nurses' faces and in their actions were truly beautiful and so inspiring, showing us how much they loved my father.

Our family took turns talking to, hugging, and kissing Dad, even though he was not conscious. We believed he heard us deep in his spirit.

Michelle, the nurse Dad loved most, came rushing in, dressed in casual jeans and top, with tears streaming down her face. Unbeknownst to us, a staff member had contacted her on her day off, knowing how close she was to Dad. He lit up every time she came in. She had such a compassionate heart and did special things for him, even cutting his hair. She could get him to sit in a chair when no one else could.

Now we hugged and cried together. She tenderly hugged and kissed Dad and spent time talking with us and discussing his grave condition. I was comforted knowing she'd be back on duty the next morning.

Later that night, Dad grew very restless. His legs moved in spasms, as if he wanted to get up and go.

The next morning the nursing staff were astounded to see Dad awake. Michelle was right there giving him porridge for breakfast. Later that morning, she had Dad sitting in a chair. Then she got him to his feet to walk a while, which he couldn't do prior to the stroke! Mum arrived and couldn't believe her eyes. She spent the whole day with her beloved husband, holding hands, laughing and kissing.

Days later Michelle confided to me, "I did a bad thing." She added with a twinkle in her eyes. "I prayed and asked God not to take your dad before Christmas. And He didn't!"

I could see by her expression that she was wondering if it was wrong to pray to keep him there in such a hopeless condition.

I smiled and hugged her. Then I assured her. "We prayed the very same thing. God heard our prayers."

~Sandra L. Hickman

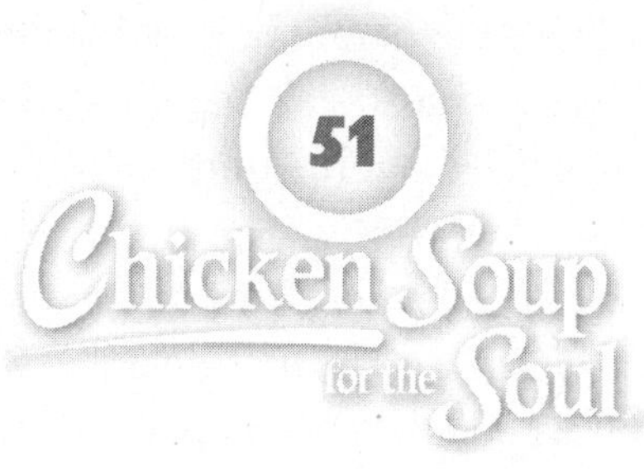

Being a Hospital Mom

As a mother comforts her child, so I will comfort you; and you will be comforted over Jerusalem.
~Isaiah 66:13 NIV

Chris was one of "my kids" on pediatrics. His foghorn voice would ring out during report and announce who he wanted to be his nurse that day. If I made out the assignments, I'd care for him, or ask others if I could be his nurse. His joy made tough days better. We laughed and talked and if I had extra time I spent it with him.

Chris had a lot of difficulty walking because of his physical handicaps. When I went on errands, I pulled him in a red wagon. He talked to everyone along the way, gave directions to new families, and made sure everybody in the hospital knew who he was, from the administrators to the housekeepers. Once he learned your name he never forgot it. He would call for staff by name, and explain exactly what he wanted from them. He had learned that to survive long periods of time in the hospital he had to demand attention, and he was rarely disappointed.

He was a charmer in every sense of the word. He fluttered his eyelashes and smiled when he asked for something, and he frowned during blood draws and procedures. He remembered everything we ever told him and repeated it to us word for word, so we learned to choose our words carefully.

Once Chris hid from me before he was due for a treatment. After twenty minutes, I was about to call the security guards to help me find him when he jumped from the linen closet.

"Boo! Surprise!"

Relieved, first I hugged him... and then started yelling at him. "Christopher! Don't you ever do that again! I was so worried that something had happened to you!" It was not one of my prouder moments as a competent nurse. After I regained my composure I told him just how worried I'd been and how sad I would be if he were hurt or lost.

That's when he began calling me Hospital Mom because I loved him enough to yell at him, just like his mom did at home.

As pediatric nurses we often do many of the "Mom" things for chronically ill kids whose parents can't be there all the time. We help the kids brush their teeth, wipe their bottoms and read them bedtime stories or make up our own. We create memories and try to make their illnesses less of a burden for them and their families. We borrow them for a time and love them when no one else can be there.

Unfortunately, Chris was on borrowed time. He had gone for a bone marrow transplant he knew was unsuccessful.

He casually said to me, "Jesus came to me and asked if I was ready to come to heaven."

I tried not to look surprised.

"I told Jesus that I would be soon, but Grandma and Mom aren't ready yet." He asked, "Kathy, do you think my mom and Grandma will see me in heaven?"

"Chris, I think they will feel you are there, but I don't know if they will be able to see you. I do think you can look down and see them, though."

I reminded him of the children he had known who were already there, and said I was sure they would be there waiting when it was his time.

"Do you think people are still sick in heaven?"

"No, I don't think so, Chris. I think heaven is the most beautiful place you can think of, and sickness is gone and love is all around you. That's heaven."

Shortly thereafter, Chris got weaker and his voice grew silent. His stepfather and I sat at his bedside and held his hand when he took his last breath.

And I cried like a mom.

~Kathleen E. Jones

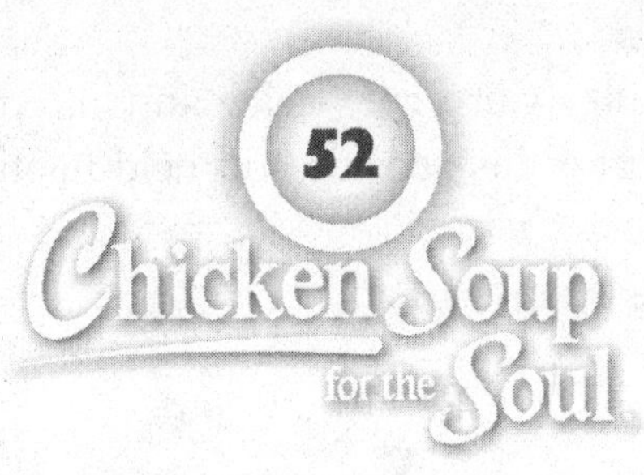

Brittany

Children are God's apostles sent forth day by day to preach of love, hope and peace.
~J.R. Lowell

I met Brittany during August at third grade registration. When she and her mother came into my office, Brittany had a scarf on her head and could barely keep her eyes open. I immediately assessed she would be too sick for school.

I explained to her mother that I would begin the paperwork for homebound care.

"She will NOT be homebound!" her mother declared.

Brittany's mom explained her daughter's very aggressive form of brain cancer. She admitted that Brittany was unable to do third grade work, but said she would spend time in the classroom just the same.

Fortunately, her compassionate teacher let Brittany do whatever work she could handle, and after a couple of hours she'd come to my clinic to rest. She would tell me stories about her three sisters and living in the country, and I'd tell her about my disobedient dog's antics.

When she was able, I'd walk with her, though she was often unsteady. When I walked too fast, she'd pull my hand. "Slow down," she'd giggle, making me laugh too. "Take your time," she coaxed.

As the year went on, Brittany's health deteriorated, but she continued to come to school. Some days she just slept in my clinic, where everyone fell in love with her. Staff members dropped by and sat with her during their breaks. Teachers bought her trinkets. The art teacher and Brittany swapped jokes. She became family.

The next year she came to school but she couldn't walk and rarely went to class. Instead, she came to the clinic and stayed as long as her little body could tolerate. It was so difficult seeing her at this stage, but it also felt right having her at school. She always wanted to hear about my dog and she gave me advice on training him.

Our favorite conversations were about angels. Brittany was fascinated by them; her sunken face lit up when she shared stories from her imagination and declared her absolute belief in them.

In September Brittany fell into a coma. When I went to see her, I knew it would be the last time. I sat by her bedside and talked as if she were with me at school, regaling her with stories of my disobedient dog. She reached for my hand.

The next day Brittany awoke briefly and told her mother, "It's time to go home. Two angels are waiting for me."

Now I feel Brittany watching over me from heaven, giggling and telling me, "Slow down!" She's still reminding me to take my time, for life is too precious to speed through.

~Nancy Mapes

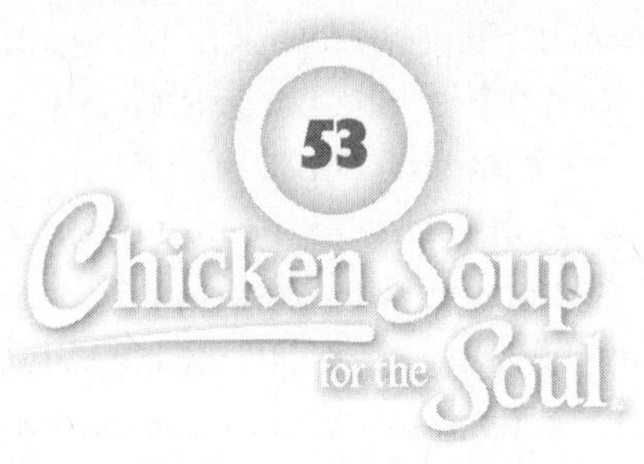

A Thank You from Heaven

Nothing is or can be accidental with God.
~Henry Wadsworth Longfellow

My wife, Kenzie, is a Licensed Practical Nurse. She worked in a group home with adults who were severely limited, both physically and cognitively. Yet these residents were sweeter than a ten-gallon tub of frosting. These were truly remarkable individuals who epitomized resiliency and strength. Sadly, they remained prisoners of their bodies. Wheelchair-bound, they were limited in mobility and speech, yet Kenzie found creative ways to communicate and interact with them.

Although the nurses weren't allowed to have "favorites," Poncho definitely pulled at Kenzie's heartstrings. He was lovably ornery, and although he was a very caring person, he gladly fulfilled the role of "grumpy old man." Kenzie knew better. Poncho was a teddy bear of a human being, and she loved and cared for him like he was her own grandfather.

Poncho eventually passed away. It was bittersweet. God knows a brave soul such as Poncho had earned respite in Heaven. Still, those who cared for him would miss him dearly, especially Kenzie. She knew he deserved a rest break on the Other Side after a long and difficult life riddled with health problems, but she grieved his loss and missed him desperately.

A few weeks after his passing, she had a dream about Poncho. In it he appeared vibrant, youthful, and healthy, not confined to a wheelchair. He smiled at Kenzie, exuding warmth and kindness. He was at peace. Perfect. He radiated a light that shone from within. Although he didn't utter a single word, Poncho embraced her in a loving hug, as if to say, "Thank you." She woke from the dream in tears, blanketed with joy.

Kenzie wiped her eyes and rolled over to look at the alarm clock on our nightstand. It read 3:17 a.m. Exhaling a breath of both grief and elation, Kenzie knew she'd had a heavenly rendezvous with the spirit of her old friend. Poncho's birthday was March 17th.

~Andy Myers

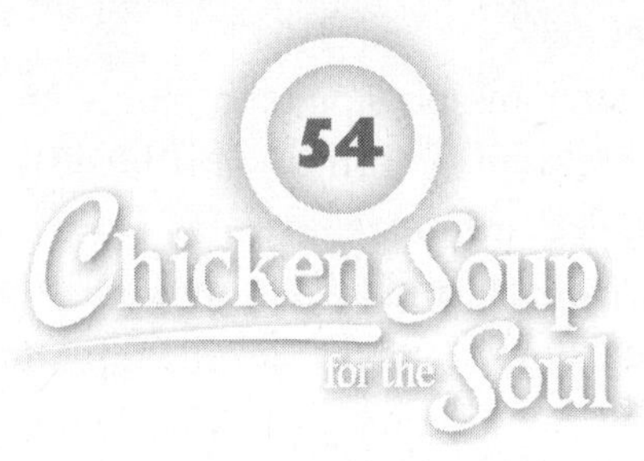

I Am a Nurse and I See Spirits

God made Truth with many doors to welcome every believer who knocks on them.
~Kahlil Gibran

I have a bachelor's degree in Nursing and a master's in Religious Psychology. I am a registered nurse and an ordained minister. And I see spirits. I prefer to think of them as angels. Whether it's a gift or curse, I think I inherited it from my father's mother.

My grandmother used to talk to bullfrogs and hummingbirds. On the morning my father died, his spirit visited her hundreds of miles away. At the moment my mother discovered Dad's body, Grandmother said she heard his voice behind her. That was my first experience with anything I would consider odd.

Naturally, as a teenager, I was not going to believe in such things. It just wasn't cool. It wasn't until years later, after I became a nurse, that I began to have unusual experiences. The moment my first patient died my eyes flew up to the corner of the room. I realized I saw the person's soul leave his body. Naturally, I never told anyone.

Over the years my favorite place was the terminal children's ward. Yes, it was heartbreaking to watch the children in pain and the suffering of their families. However, the children inspired me. They could see angels and they were not afraid to talk about them to anyone who would listen. One small blind child told me she could see an angel named Candle and that Candle was there to help her die. Although too weak to move her mortal body, I could see her reach up and take the hand of her angel and smile.

Over the years I witnessed the dying process over and over. If not for the time spent with the children I would have become deeply depressed. Because of them I remained hopeful as my experiences expanded. I could sense a spirit hovering as we worked to revive a critical patient. I could see a puff, a mist, which I knew was the soul leaving as a person let out his last breath.

One evening, in the emergency room, a seventeen-year-old boy was brought in with chest pains. He'd been playing in a church basketball game when he collapsed. He was placed in one of the two glass rooms directly across from the desk where I sat using the computer. He was alert and talking while being given a full cardiac work-up.

A few minutes later, a trauma was called. EMS came rushing in with another seventeen-year-old who had sustained multiple gunshot wounds to the chest while committing an armed felony. He was placed in the glass room to the left of the first boy. The trauma team went to work on him and, although they didn't expect him to make it to surgery, the surgery team was notified.

Even though the first boy couldn't see what was going on next door, he started praying out loud for that person's life to be spared. It was then that I saw the death angel. He looked just like the many pictures I had seen but without the sickle. Then I saw the young basketball player close his eyes and lie back. His spirit came out of his body and stood between the death angel and the other boy. I clearly heard his words. "Take me in his place. I am ready."

Just as all three vanished, the cardiac monitor alarmed and straight-lined. Instantly the code team was in the room working on the young basketball player. All the emergency heart equipment, code cart and medications were already at his bedside. His cardiac specialist was right there at the desk. He should have made it, but he didn't. The young criminal with multiple gunshot wounds should not have made it, but he did.

I, like the other workers in the emergency room, was stunned. I wasn't about to tell anyone what I had seen. However, when I was asked to minister to the grieving family of the young basketball player I found myself telling them what I saw. The mother listened intently and she actually smiled. "Thank you," she said. "Just before you came in, I was asking God why. Why He took a boy as good as my son, so young. He sent my answer through you."

Now you see why I rarely tell these stories. I'm a nurse, and I see spirits.

~Debbie Sistare

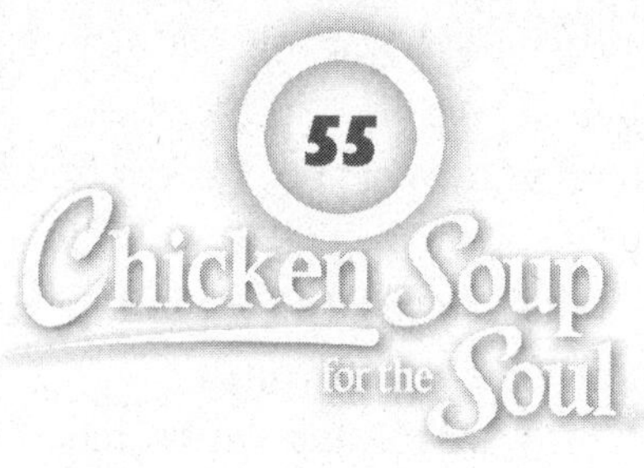

Buttercup

Every flower is a soul blossoming in nature.
~Gérard de Nerval

Val couldn't help but be a favorite patient on the palliative care unit where I worked. She was the happiest, most positive person I'd ever known. We developed a special connection and joked with each other about everything.

When I told her that my son was getting married, she wanted to see pictures of my dress. I brought in a picture of the long electric-blue strapless gown I had chosen.

"Brenda," she said, "that's the most beautiful dress I've ever seen. And you will look even more beautiful wearing it. You'll have to bring in photos of the wedding and tell me all about it."

"I promise," I said, as I clasped her hand, hoping she would still be around to see them, because despite her cheery disposition, we both knew she was dying.

Over the next few weeks, Val's health deteriorated. Instead of helping her get to the washroom so she could bathe herself, I was now washing her in bed. But rather than be upset, Val simply saw it as more time for us to visit and share. I told her about the new house my husband and I were moving into and I promised her more pictures.

Even on days Val wasn't assigned to me, I always made a point of going to see her and giving her a hug. "Morning, Sunshine," I'd say. "Just came to say hello."

"Oh Brenda, that's so nice of you. I know how busy all you nurses are."

I grinned. "Val, you know I'd never miss a chance to see you. It brightens my day just being with you."

Once she leaned toward me and whispered, "Don't tell the others, but you're one of my favorite nurses."

I whispered back. "Don't tell anyone, but you're one of my favorite patients." Warmth flooded my heart.

Some days later, while I was bathing her, we spoke on a more serious note.

"Now that I've gotten a bit better, I'm planning to go back to my retirement home."

"Oh, Val," I joked, "don't tell me you're getting tired of me already."

She smiled. "No, but it's time to go home for a while. I know I'll be back here again and that I won't be leaving the next time. At least not for the retirement home."

For a moment I didn't say anything. We both knew it was the truth.

Then I realized I did have one more service to offer her. "When you do come back here, you may not know me or be conscious, but I will know you and I promise to take extra special care of you."

She nodded and took a deep breath, then touched my hand. "It makes me feel good knowing I have a friend in the hospital."

Val did indeed get better and went back to her retirement home. Weeks later I visited her there. She'd lost all her hair and was now wearing a wig, but she was the same Val. We talked for a while, then she got tired and it was time for me to leave.

"Next time you come," she said, "we'll have a glass of wine in the bar. No sense living in a swanky place if you can't have a drink or two with friends."

Unfortunately, before we could have that drink, Val returned to our palliative care unit. My shift had ended, but just as I was about to leave I saw her lying on a stretcher without her wig. I went to her and held her hand.

A smile creased her face. "I remember your promise to take special care of me. I'm holding you to that promise."

I squeezed her hand to show that I remembered.

Over the next few weeks Val's health deteriorated, but she remained cheerful and our special connection held strong. We continued to chat about all sorts of things.

One day during her bath I asked her, "If you could be reincarnated as something, what would it be."

She replied instantly. "A buttercup."

"Not a rose?"

"Too showy," she replied. "Definitely a buttercup."

A few days later, Val fell unconscious and shortly thereafter died with her daughters beside her.

We're not supposed to get too involved with our patients, but I felt saddened over the loss of Val. While it's not remarkable for me to attend funerals if they are close, seldom do I travel to another city. But, this time I felt I had to drive those miles to honor my friend. When I arrived, I hugged her daughters and told them how much I'd miss her. They thanked me for caring for their mom, but I told them it had been a privilege.

On the return trip home, I pulled into the driveway of our new house. As I walked to the front door, I surveyed my newly acquired garden that was already growing well in May. I noted the purple irises blooming, and then something caught my eye. I looked closer and there amid the other plants was a splash of yellow.

A buttercup.

~Brenda Dickie

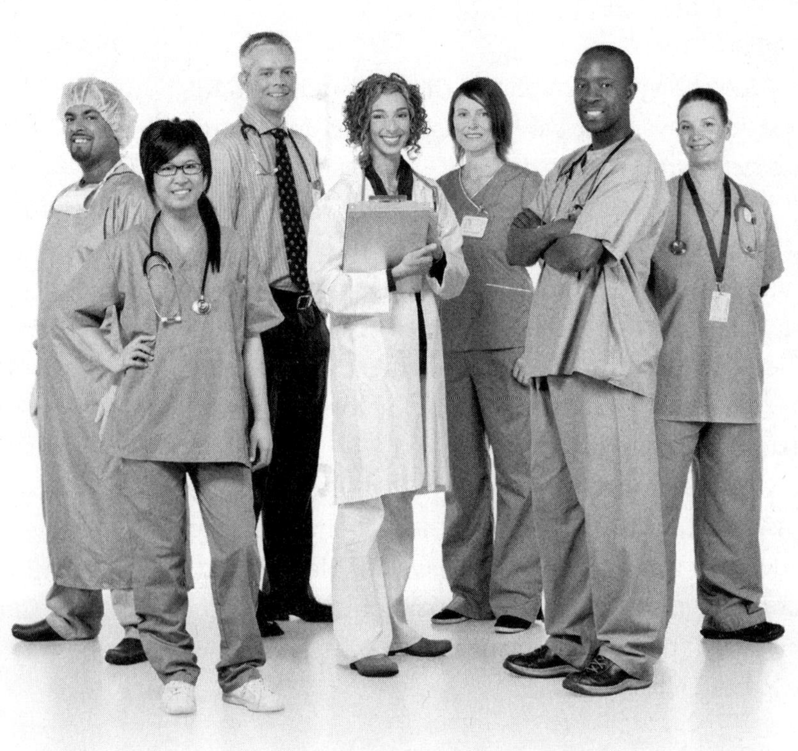

Inspiration for Nurses

Angels Among Us

Believers, look up — take courage. The angels are nearer than you think.

~Billy Graham

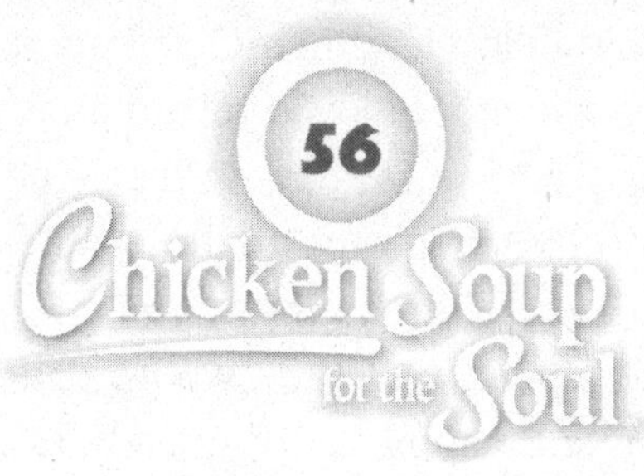

Playing with Angels

We pass now quickly from each other's sight; but I know full well that where beyond these passing scenes you shall be, there will be Heaven.
~Joshua Chamberlain

The first time I walked in his room, I knew there was something special about him. Taking care of him always made my day.

Connor was only six months old when he was diagnosed with acute myeloid leukemia (AML). He spent the next nine months in the hospital. Whether I was administering painful steroid eye drops, or drawing blood from his central line, he smiled at me behind his pacifier. All the nurses were ecstatic when we heard he would receive a bone marrow transplant from his sister, a perfect match.

After his transplant, he stayed in a Ronald McDonald house for six months until he was deemed stable enough to go home. Shortly after, Connor's mother noticed a lump behind his ear and took him to the doctor. A biopsy revealed a relapse of AML. Connor had to gear up for a new, more intense round of chemotherapy, which would hopefully be followed by another bone marrow transplant from an unrelated donor.

Throughout everything, Connor always kept that smile that could brighten any room. When he came back to us he still had that smile, but by then he could talk. Hearing him say my name with his sweet voice made my heart melt. He loved to run around the unit chasing nurses, chasing his sister, and riding on his IV pole with his dad. To say he was a happy child would be an understatement. And that was his mother's goal, to keep him happy.

His family had agreed that they would continue treatments as long as Connor was still happy. Unfortunately, after several rounds of chemotherapy, a missed window for bone marrow transplant due to a sick donor, and another relapse, he was out of options. Seven months from his initial relapse, Connor went home on hospice.

Sometimes, as a pediatric oncology nurse, it is easier to imagine that these kids go home and have some sort of miracle. So if we never see them again we can pretend it's because they are still living and growing up, playing with their friends, going to school, like every kid should. Connor, however, came back to us. His parents decided it would be too traumatizing for his sister if he died at home.

When he first came back, he slept most of the time. The doctors figured he had about a week left. One week turned into two, and Connor continued to amaze everyone. After sleeping for days, he would wake up and want to play. He wouldn't play alone, though. He told his mom, "Look, look!" and he giggled and smiled with his new friend that only he could see. "An angel!"

This continued for almost three weeks. Connor would sleep for a couple of days, and then wake up and play with angels for a few hours before going back to sleep. I watched in amazement as this little boy taught me about faith.

One night, as I took care of Connor, his breathing worsened, his color changed, and his alertness decreased significantly. At the family's request, I called the chaplain at 11:00 p.m. They asked if I could stay in the room. My coworkers encouraged me to do so, even taking over the rest of my patient load so I could provide support to this very special family.

We sat and talked all night. We laughed about our favorite Connor memories. We cried, thinking about a future without this beautiful child. His mom said she knew I loved Connor. His parents expressed their impending grief and fear of the unknown. They told me, however, about their undying faith, and their certainty that their son was about to become an angel, welcomed into heaven.

The hours passed, and at 7:00 a.m., it was time for me to give shift report. I told the family and the chaplain I would be back to say goodbye before heading home. As I started to give report to the day shift nurse, I looked over, and Connor's dad was waving in the window for me to come back in the room.

I sprinted as fast as I could to see Connor awake, waving and yelling out, "Bye!" He looked right at me, waved, and said, "Bye!" He gazed at each person in the room… his mom, his dad, his sister, the chaplain… waved to each and said, "Bye!"

His parents then lay down in bed next to him and he turned to look at his dad. His dad kissed him and said, "It's okay. You can go, you can go. I love you, I love you, I love you." Connor touched his face, and then turned and looked at his mom. She kissed him and then whispered to him, "I love you, I love you. I will see you again. You can go, I love you." And with that, he touched his mom's face, lay on his back, and passed away.

As the entire room burst into tears, there was an unspoken certainty that we just witnessed something truly amazing. Connor was playing with the angels again.

~Molly K.

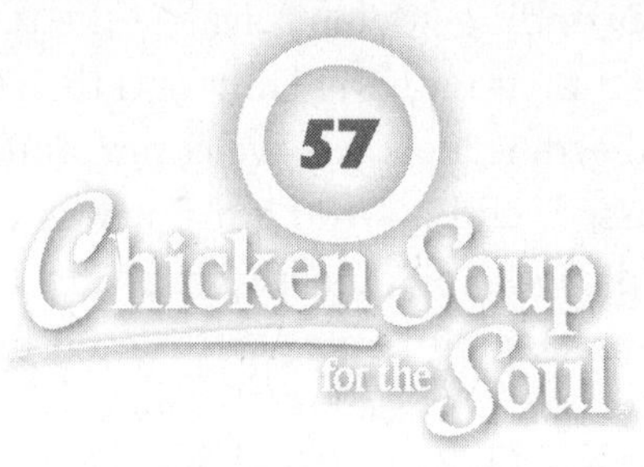

Angel in India

The human body has limitations. The human spirit is boundless.
~Dean Karnazes

In the midst of a grueling, five-year stint at medical school, I was invited to volunteer at a health camp in India for a few weeks and I accepted without hesitation. I was joined by volunteers from many NGOs.

Our journey started in Bangalore, and included several exhausting hours of a bus ride on a dusty bumpy road. When we finally reached the village at 8:00 p.m., it was pouring rain and the roads were ankle-deep in mud.

We started our activities the next morning, and in a week's time most of us felt like we'd been there forever. But as our trip drew to a close, I was sorry I was leaving.

On the eve of our departure, I began feeling a little uneasy, and at dinner the room suddenly started whirling around me. A fellow volunteer put her palm to my forehead and gasped. I was running a fever of 104 degrees Fahrenheit. Because there was a spurt of dengue cases that year, I decided to get tested. My blood sample was sent to the only lab around, fifty kilometers away. At midnight, we found out I had dengue hemorrhagic fever.

Over the next few hours my symptoms worsened. My fever spiked, I had a headache that felt like my skull was splitting in two, and my bones felt like they were breaking. No wonder dengue is also known as "break-bone fever." At 5:00 a.m., it was decided that I was too ill to stay in the village so an ambulance picked me up and took me to the hospital in a neighboring town.

When I was admitted and placed in a tiny room on the top floor of the hospital, I understood what it meant to be truly alone. My parents were thousands of miles away, my boyfriend was at a conference in Vienna, and all the people I knew were scheduled to leave in a few hours. Some volunteers offered to cancel their tickets and stay with me, but I didn't want to ruin their plans, so I refused.

So there I was, all alone, in a strange room in a strange place, too weak and nauseated to even sit up, and running a temperature so high my brain felt like it would melt. A nurse came in to take my temperature. From the look on her face I could tell it wasn't good news. At that moment, I couldn't take it anymore, and I broke down, sobbing. The nurse, Maya, put her arms around me. She was around fifty, with graying hair and soft kind eyes. She reminded me of my mom and immediately I felt comforted. She reached for my hand and squeezed it.

It was as if we had entered a pact, as from that moment on, Sister Maya was always there when I opened my eyes. When the bouts of nausea and vomiting began, she was there to hold my hair back for me. She then made me sip water with a teaspoon so I would stay hydrated, all the while gently stroking my forehead. When my platelet count dropped to a dangerous 30,000 and I was bleeding from my nose into my eyes and urine, Sister Maya hovered, examining me every fifteen minutes for new signs of bleed, in case I needed a platelet transfusion. Because I had to be pricked every six hours to monitor my platelet count, all the veins in my arms were painfully swollen, and when they decided to draw blood through a vein on my foot, Sister Maya held me tightly as I howled in pain. When my hands throbbed excruciatingly from the intravenous cannula, she massaged them for hours, gently breaking the clots that had formed in the vessels. When I was too weak to get up on my own, she carried me to the bathroom.

One night, fluid started collecting in my lungs and abdomen and every breath was painful. Sister Maya propped me up and whispered comfortingly about how I would soon get better and how I had to hang in there. When my blood pressure dipped to dangerously low levels and I had to be shifted to the ICU, Sister Maya held my hand and never left my side, even cancelling her regular shifts and staying with me for more than twenty-four hours at a stretch.

When I took this turn for the worse, my folks were informed. But given my condition, I feared I wouldn't last until they came. In med school, I had read about the innumerable complications of dengue fever and the high fatality rates, but until that moment, I had never realized how terrifying it could be.

When I cried out of fear, Sister Maya held my hand and prayed with me, for me. She begged me to have faith, to never lose hope, and to be strong enough to fight this illness. For hours, while I slipped in and out of consciousness, she sat next to me, her hand never leaving mine, whispering prayers and words of encouragement in my ear.

On the third morning, Sister Maya had an idea. She had once read that freshly squeezed juice of raw papaya leaves helped raise platelet counts. She contacted a friend who brought it in for me. When I tasted the intensely bitter green liquid, I gagged, but Sister Maya coaxed me to finish the dose. After two more doses in the afternoon and night, she sat with her fingers crossed and her head bowed in prayer as my platelet counts were being reassessed in the lab.

When I opened my eyes at 5:00 the next morning, I had a pleasant surprise. My platelets had risen to 64,000 and my condition was stable enough for me to be moved out of the ICU. I put my arms around Sister Maya and we both cried with joy.

When my parents arrived that evening, I was strong enough to sit up and smile at them. Slowly, I started getting better, and a week later I was discharged. It took me four weeks to fight off the illness completely. When I think of those dark days, I shudder to think I almost gave up, and I smile to think of the angel who helped me fight.

It's been two years now, and I plan to go back and visit Sister Maya later this year. She instilled in me a profound respect for nurses, and more importantly, a staunch belief in the healing power of the human spirit that they deliver.

~Pallavi Kamat

My Greatest Help

When you become detached mentally from yourself and concentrate on helping other people with their difficulties, you will be able to cope with your own more effectively.
~Norman Vincent Peale

I stood in the middle of my living room looking up toward the heavens. "God, I need a miracle and I need one now."

At that exact moment, the phone rang. "This is Beth. I'm a registered nurse with your health insurance company. I coach our members who have chronic back pain."

Her voice was like a soothing balm. I knew immediately she was the answer to my prayer.

It had been three years since my back surgery, since my life had changed so drastically. Once a very active person, I didn't know how to live in this broken body. Nobody had been able to help me. All the doctors and physical therapists left me feeling hopeless. I had gone to many medical professionals and they had no answers for me.

Then Beth came into my life. We clicked instantly. She told me she would be calling me once a week and we'd chat for thirty minutes. I really needed her encouragement in my life because I couldn't see anything positive. It was one of my lowest points ever.

After my surgery, I had flare-ups when I pushed myself too hard. They would put me in bed for months. It didn't take much. If I walked a little too long, or did too much housework, or sat in the car for an extended period of time, I developed crippling pain.

Beth taught me how to listen to my body. She asked me what my pain level was on a scale of one to ten. If it was over three, I had done too much and I needed to stop and rest. Resting wasn't something I was used to doing. I learned not only how to pace myself physically, but to change the way I thought about things.

I had felt useless because I wasn't the woman I used to be, but Beth taught me how to be thankful for the things I could do and to celebrate myself. That's something I had never done in a healthy body, so this was healing for me on a deep level.

Every week she had a different lesson for me to work on. One week I wrote down all of my positive attributes. Another, all the nice things and compliments anyone had ever said to me. I also wrote all the things I liked about myself. Beth said, "Meditate on these things." What an eye opening experience for me!

I'd always thought if I couldn't be everything to everybody, I was a failure. But I learned from our sessions about my inherent strength and potential.

When I was invited to my godson's wedding, I didn't know how I would be able to sit through the whole ceremony. I was worried about letting his family down when Beth said, "Don't you think they'll be happy that you were able to attend? It doesn't matter how long you can stay." Her voice was so friendly and cheerful that whenever she corrected my thinking, it put me at ease. She had a way of putting everything in perspective for me.

I thought she must have such a contented life; she always sounded so happy. I could hear her smile through the phone. Her joy became my strength for those thirty minutes.

As time went by, I got to know her better. She shared that her husband and only son were both disabled. I was shocked. She lived with challenges most people will never experience. Her burdens were far more difficult than mine, yet she gave pure joyfulness to all her patients.

After several weeks of talking on the phone, I asked her if she would like to meet me for lunch. I waited outside the café and when

I noticed someone walking down the street with a bounce in her step and a smile on her face, I knew it had to be Beth. We hugged each other warmly and had a wonderful time together.

We met for lunch periodically for several years. One day, I asked, "How are you always so happy and giving considering the hardships and personal challenges you face in your own life?"

She said, "I love my job and put all my trust in God."

Then I told her that, by coincidence, I had been talking to God right before she called me that first time. I said, "You must have a direct line to him to have answered my call so quickly. You helped manage my pain and my life. I had just prayed for a miracle, and you delivered."

~Marijo Herndon

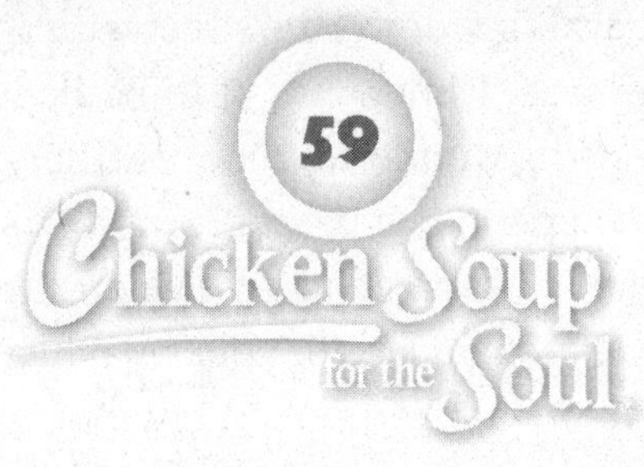

The Gold Miners

Too often we underestimate the power of a touch, a smile, a kind word, a listening ear, an honest compliment, or the smallest act of caring, all of which have the potential to turn a life around.
~Leo Buscaglia

I struggled with mental health issues for most of my life. Growing up I thought I was just odd but in my late twenties I decided that something was wrong and I needed help. I started off with a therapist, then another one, added some drugs to the mix and finally went into the hospital for a lengthy assessment.

My time there was not well spent. Fear left me almost mute and the new pills they gave me did nothing for me but make me fat. On that rare occasion when I absolutely had to speak I would choose a nurse carefully. By watching and listening I figured out who might be safe. Trust came hard for me so talking to anyone required an indescribable amount of grit. Some nurses viewed this selection process as favoritism. Of course I had favorites, just like I had favorite teachers in school and favorite pajamas. Why would I speak with someone who pushed too hard or judged without understanding? I needed to be understood.

Once someone decided it would be good for me to have a student follow me around for a few days a week. It was a strange choice considering the fact that I never spoke. What would the student learn?

Fortunately there was a nurse I had identified as being "safe." For the first time, I spoke up. I went to her and while studying my shoes I told her how I felt about having a student.

"Then you don't have to have one." She just smiled and I walked away feeling as if I had passed a test. I had talked and somebody had listened.

Over time there were many visits to the hospital, as doctors tried to find the right pills, a proper diagnosis, and a treatment plan. With each admission new faces replaced old ones and I would have to evaluate the new people. Once, when I went down to the nurse's station to see who came on shift, a new person was sitting there. I was told that I would be her patient. But I wanted a nurse who I knew. I scowled and she just kept smiling. I almost stomped my feet as I headed back to my room.

This "scowl–smile" form of communication went on for a few days. Then one night this nurse dropped in to see how I was doing. I was very sad about something. Lo and behold I talked! I have no memory of the words I used, but when I was finished she didn't push for me to go further. Instead she asked if I could use a hug and I shocked myself by saying yes. This was huge for me.

Bedtimes were difficult and long after other patients were fast asleep I stayed hyper vigilant. I would read or write in my journal, occasionally drawing stick people. Late one night the nurse who had hugged me dropped in for a visit. Coffee in hand, she plunked herself down in the visitor's chair. And we talked. Not really about my issues, as I still had little insight into them, but about everyday things. She laughed at some of my dryly-expressed observations on life.

This coffee talk became a ritual when she worked nights. It helped me so much. She wasn't trying to pry me open and our interactions made me feel valued as a human being. If I said something that she found to be unacceptable, I received a light reprimand, but not very often. Eventually she would finish her coffee, give me a hug and wander off to do paperwork.

During one of my early admissions it was acknowledged that a high level of anxiety was what left me tongue-tied. It also left me with a need for solitude. If I got stuck with a roommate, I found great places to hide around the hospital. Everyone who worked with me assumed that I was an introvert. When things were good I could talk the ears off a deaf donkey, but then I would be discharged, so the staff seldom saw this extroverted side of me. It was as if there was a me who laughed and talked and a me who shut down, leaving everyone around me puzzled and concerned. Switching between these selves meant another admission to a hospital room with yellow blankets and shower curtains that clung to me like live snakes.

I met a male nurse after one shift change. His wife had actually been my therapist for a short time. I didn't talk to her either. By this time though, I had begun to find my voice. As with the Coffee Cup Nurse, the man would drop by to see me after the other patients were settled. Nurse Husband spoke to me kindly and with respect, as if he were searching for things that would draw me out. One night he began to talk about children's developmental stages. He brought a textbook in, pointing out one particular theorist, and left it with me.

I read it with a keen sense of interest and I talked about it eagerly the next evening. I discussed each section, reciting incidents that would have caused part of me to become stuck in each emotional stage. It was actually one of the most interesting conversations I had during my stays. Being treated like a normal intelligent person was like putting a stake in the ground to mark a spot from which I could make progress.

When I wasn't in the hospital, I worked with a therapist. That hard work with her was combined with the help of the nurses who viewed me as an intelligent person, I opened up more and more. I started to find my way past the walls I had erected around myself. In time, I gained enough control over my peaks and valleys that I was able to work on myself without further need of hospitalization.

The work helped me to realize what caused my fear and withdrawal. I have Dissociative Identity Disorder, formerly known as Multiple Personality Disorder. Receiving that book from Nurse Husband was a turning point. It explained that various traumas left part of me stuck in each of Erikson's stages of growth. That was how I had become "we." It was because of this condition that I could rarely speak, having been trained not to talk or trust.

Many professionals have helped me to understand my world in order to gain more control over it. Without the nurses who saw past my games of emotional hide and seek, I truly believe it would have taken me a lot longer to reach the level of awareness I have today.

The trust I developed allowed me to retrain myself with guidance from many people. Among them were determined nurses who were like gold miners, never giving up until they uncovered the parts of me that could shake off the dust and shine.

~Catherine Hannah Grey

A Gift of Sun

Kindness in words creates confidence. Kindness in thinking creates profoundness. Kindness in giving creates love.
~Lao Tzu

I suffer from Seasonal Affective Disorder, so every year the start of spring signals my freedom from the gloomy imprisonment of winter despair. One year, on the very first day of spring, I was relishing the sun on my walk from work to my favorite lunch spot. The sun radiated its warmth on my shoulders and the birds were singing in the trees. I was twenty-seven years old and happy to be free of the dark, icy winter months. But, all of a sudden, I felt scorching pain in my abdomen. It turned out that an unknown tumor on my liver had ruptured.

During the next months, I trudged from walk-in clinic to CT scan to oncologist to interventional radiologist to surgeon, fighting the tumor with all the weapons of modern medicine. I spent hours, days, and weeks in waiting rooms, exam rooms, and hospital rooms with no windows, and therefore, no sun.

After waking from my final surgery, a resection in which forty-five percent of my liver was removed, I was terrified: terrified that maybe some of the tumor still clung to my liver, terrified by the horrendous fog of the general anesthesia, terrified of the pain that far exceeded the rupture itself, terrified that I did not know where I was, but mostly terrified to be alone there in the recovery area. My parents lived far away and my surgery was performed on a Monday, a day all my friends needed to be at work.

When Mary-Jean, the nurse tending to me, asked if I had any family in the waiting room, I told her — with words that shot stabbing pains up my abdomen — that I did not.

Mary-Jean then asked if she could get anything for me. What I craved first and foremost was water, but the doctor's orders dictated I couldn't have that yet, not even ice chips. And so, in my bewildered haze, I asked instead for three things.

The first was calming classical music.

The second was *The Little Prince*, a childhood favorite that my father often read to me as a child.

The third thing I asked for? Some sun.

I now remember this with some embarrassment. There I was, an adult supporting myself in a difficult city, regressed into a child. I was asking the impossible of Mary-Jean, someone who had several other patients in equally dire straits, someone who had been working for hours rushing from patient to patient with what I can only imagine were aching feet, someone who had never met me and had no obligation to care about my plight beyond getting me the right medications and taking my vitals. On top of that, I hadn't brought headphones to listen to music, and I certainly did not have a copy of *The Little Prince* with me.

"I'll try my best," she said, gently and without even a dash of annoyance. She recommended that I sleep if I could, and assured me that while I was sleeping, she would come by every ten minutes to press the button that would flood my system with fentanyl and keep my pain at bay, so the pain wouldn't wake me, and so that when I woke up, it would not be to a shock of agony. I thanked her with the fewest but most heartfelt words I could. "When I get out of here, I'd like to write you a long thank-you note."

When I woke, Mary-Jean came by to see how I was doing. She touched my arm as a mother might, with comfort, while she took my vitals. "I remember what you asked for," she said, though I barely remembered myself what I had requested. Then Mary-Jean introduced me to another nurse, a woman around my age named Kara, who cared for me during the brief time that Mary-Jean took her lunch break.

Mary-Jean came back in what seemed to be a fraction of a minute, but whether that was because the fentanyl had rearranged my sense of time or because her lunch "hour" was so short, I did not know. I asked her how her lunch was, only imagining the difficulty of working long shifts with short breaks to gobble down some food. "It was a great success," she told me.

Then, like a magician, like Mary Poppins, like a loving parent, she pulled out two objects from a plastic bag: a pair of headphones and a paperback copy of *The Little Prince*. "And," she said, "I've made a special request that you'll be brought to a corner room with plenty of light."

I write this now from my writing desk at home, at the same desk where I wrote Mary-Jean that thank-you note I promised: a letter of gratitude over three pages long. On a shelf just above my desk, I keep those headphones and that copy of *The Little Prince* that Mary-Jean brought to me in my greatest moment of vulnerability. I look at them every day, and when I do, I remember the tremendous kindness that exists deep within the core of people like Mary-Jean: a force so beautiful that it brought me the sun.

~Flora Dash

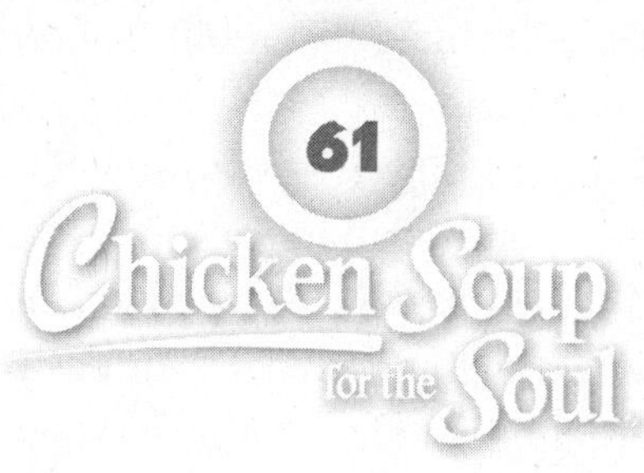

Never Underestimate an Army Nurse

I came to realize that life lived to help others is the only one that matters and that it is my duty. This is my highest and best use as a human.

~Ben Stein

I don't remember her name. I don't even remember a clear picture of her face. In my mind's eye all I see is the outline of an Army nurse. I see the short-sleeved, pale green uniform top with the shadows of epaulets on her shoulders. The cut of her A-line skirt. Her stockinged legs from the knees down, and the sturdy brown shoes on her feet. I see the crisp pleat in the center of the back of her shirt. And the small half moons of sweat in her armpits. She is clearest to me from behind because it was from that position that she played such a big role in my life.

I am the fifth of ten children. My mother drank. When she was at her worst, we got shipped out to relatives. I got shipped out on repeated occasions to stay with my mother's youngest sister. My aunt's family consisted of her son, who was six months younger than I, and her Army officer husband. Every time I went to stay with them I got to sleep in a bedroom fit for a princess, with a canopy bed, a vanity table, and a dresser taller than I was, all in winter white wood. While it was a welcome change from the tiny bedroom I shared with my two older sisters, I never really liked that room. I never felt comfortable in it because it cost too much.

The summer I turned nine I went to stay with my aunt and her family at Fort Sam Houston, in San Antonio, Texas. Within a month of my arrival I had taught myself to hypercirculate. I learned how to raise my body temperature and give myself flash nosebleeds. I went to the emergency room a lot that summer. They thought it was the Texas heat. Or maybe an allergic reaction to something.

Late in the summer, I was taken to the emergency room once again with a gushing bloody nose. There was a new nurse on duty that day who turned around and looked me in the eyes. I don't know if she took a liking to me, or if she sensed something was up. Or maybe she had just looked at my fat and growing medical file and saw the repeat visits to the ER. Whatever it was, she was instantly kind to me. Kind and protective. She asked me what my favorite color was and what I wanted to be when I grew up. She asked me questions that had nothing to do with what was happening to me at night in my aunt's house. And then she did something no one else had thought to do: she got me admitted to the hospital.

Fear crossed my aunt's face when the nurse said I was being admitted. Her human shield would be absent from her house that night. Jealousy passed across my cousin's face. I didn't look at the face of my aunt's husband.

The nurse got me into a wheelchair and turned her back on them and wheeled me away. She pulled the curtains around me and gave me privacy to change, without my having to ask. She got me settled into bed and let me pick what I wanted for dinner. She came back with my meal tray and a short stack of books. She pulled a chair close and read to me as I ate. Dinner and the rhythmic rise and fall of her voice were the perfect lullaby for a nine-year-old black girl who had trouble sleeping.

Once I had finished my second dinner tray, the nurse helped me clean up and settle down in the bed. She started reading again from where she had left off. In the middle of the story, in the middle of a sentence, in the middle of her taking a breath to read the next word, my aunt's husband came into my hospital room.

There was no plan between the nurse and me, no signal given, no exchange of any untoward information. But the minute that door opened, I shut my eyes and let my body go limp. My ears were wide open, though. I heard the nurse shush him and tell him without skipping a beat that I was sound asleep.

He stopped so abruptly that his shoes squeaked on the hospital floor.

"Nurse," he said, and it wasn't a title of respect. "What are you doing here?"

"Keeping an eye on my patient."

"What did you say to me, Lieutenant?"

When he called her by her rank, she put the book down and stood at attention. "Sir," she said, "I am keeping an eye on my patient, Sir."

He told her he knew she wasn't still on duty.

She countered with a desire to go above and beyond the call.

He warned her that he was perfectly capable of watching his niece.

She countered with being needed in case the nosebleed recurred.

He gave her a direct order to leave my hospital room.

She stood at attention and responded, "Sir, no Sir!"

He gave the order again and again.

I couldn't see either of their faces, but I could hear the fitful rising of his anger and her robot-like parroting of that one single phrase. Her tone was one of utmost respect, and utmost resilience. She never got angry; she never got loud; and she never moved from my bedside.

He was yelling at her. You could feel the vibration of it and the pop of moisture as he spat the words in her face.

I don't know how I managed to stay still. Maybe it was something in the sureness of her refusal to leave me. If she could stand up to the man who had terrorized so many of my nights, then I could feign sleep.

He left my hospital room in a huff, calling her, in muttered exhales, all of the nasty names they reserve for women who don't do what they're told. He threatened her with all kinds of repercussions, both personal and military. And then the soft whoosh of the hospital door closing cut him off.

The nurse did not say a single thing to me about what had just happened. She simply sat back down in the chair and began to read from the book at the place where she had left off. Again her voice worked to calm me to my bones. I tipped over into blessed sleep.

For those three nights I spent in the hospital, that nurse, whoever she was, gave me the first nights of peace in my very young life. She gave me a glimpse of what it means to stand up to a bully. She never said a single word to me about what was happening to me in my aunt's home. She just gave me a few precious days of safety that showed me a world where that didn't have to happen to me. Whoever she was, wherever she is, bless her.

~Cassandra Brent

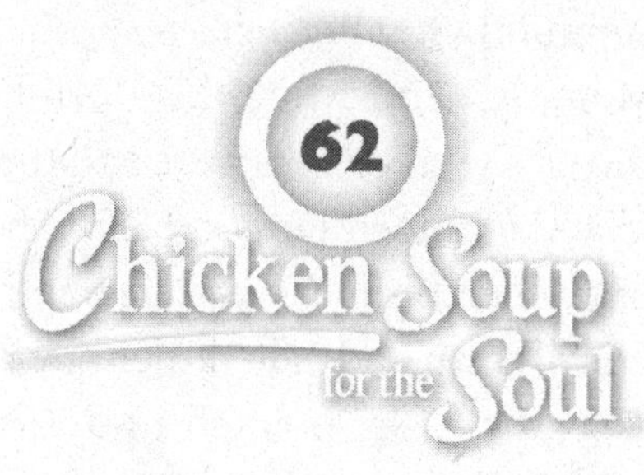

Angels in the NICU

I love these little people; and it is not a slight thing when they, who are so fresh from God, love us.
~Charles Dickens

Babies in the Neonatal Intensive Care Unit are the most innocent and precious souls on this earth. I feel pure love in their presence.

When they are having a major heart dip and oxygen drop, I whisper, "Don't go to the Light... please come back." If no one else is nearby, I may even say softly out loud, "Not on my watch, little angel." When they have those death defying color changes, I hope in my heart that they are in the arms of angels passing back and forth between this world and the other side.

There are a few nurses in our NICU who have actually seen angels. I have not seen them, but I have certainly felt their presence.

One day, as I was caring for a sick baby boy on the ventilator, his little sister came in with her mother to see her baby brother for the first time. This little girl had been a preemie in our unit four years earlier.

She was one of the most inquisitive four-year-olds I'd ever met. It was as if somewhere in her subconscious, she knew this place and wanted to know more than most siblings. Usually they are interested in seeing their baby brother or sister, and are either oblivious to the equipment or fascinated with it. This little one wanted to know about each caregiver surrounding her brother.

"Who's that, Mommy? And who's that?" And so on it went, her mom telling her who all the caregivers were and their names. Then the little sister stopped and stomped her foot. "No, that's not *everyone*!"

So I went around her brother's warmer and pointed out each member of the medical team and called them by name.

Finally, in exasperation, she pointed up to the ceiling and said, "No! Who's *that* lady? The one up there?"

She was so adamant that the embarrassed mother finally said, "Stop it. There is no one there."

But I knew. And the little sister knew. She saw her brother's guardian angel.

~Nancy J. Brooks

Good Night Nurse

Millions of spiritual creatures walk the earth unseen, both when we sleep and when we wake.
~John Milton

I don't remember much about my stay in a Dallas, Texas hospital. All day people would come and go, never breathing a word. I felt like my bed was an open casket. People peered down at me as if expecting to find a corpse.

My temperature hovered stubbornly at 103 degrees during the day, then shot up to 105 and 106 degrees at night. The doctors told me I had a life-threatening infection in my abdomen caused by a sexually transmitted disease. I felt so ashamed and dirty. My body ached like an arthritic old woman, although I'd just turned nineteen. Since sleep eluded me, I just lay in bed, terrified of dying and certain I was going to hell. I should've been fighting for my life, but I wasn't sure I wanted to live.

Enter Jean, the night nurse. She'd step into my dark room, her white uniform gleaming. As she came closer, the polyester in the fabric rustled like angel's wings. Her shoes made squeaking noises on the recently washed floor. After recording my vitals, she always leaned in close and whispered, "Still having trouble sleeping? Can I bring you a wet cloth? That forehead of yours is hotter than a Fourth of July picnic."

It took effort for me to speak. "Yes. Thank you."

Jean would disappear into the bathroom, then reappear holding comfort in her hand. "This cloth will cool you down. Do you want another gown? You're perspiring more than a West Texas field hand. I grew up on a ranch so I know what it is to sweat."

Jean would sit me up in bed and pull a clean gown over my head. For a minute, I was like a doll in her hands, but I quickly sank back in bed, too weak to properly thank her.

I considered Jean's visits my little taste of heaven since I figured I'd never go there. I couldn't see her well, though. Not because of the dim light, but because I hadn't brought my contacts to the hospital. Her face was a blur. Her white uniform and large frame gave her the appearance of being some kind of spirit floating nearby.

Jean appeared beside my bed for four days and nights. "You have beautiful hair. But it's matted to your head. How long has it been since you washed it?" I mumbled something that most likely wasn't helpful.

"My shift is over at 6:30 in the morning. How about I come back then and we'll wash that hair. You could use a shower and a new gown, too."

"I'm not sure I can stand. My legs feel like mush."

"Don't you worry. I'll make sure you don't fall. You'll feel better once you're spiffed up."

My smile was weak, but it let her know I was on board with her plan.

True to her word, Jean returned to help me down the hall to the bathroom with a shower. The huge bottle of penicillin hanging from a contraption over my bed accompanied us. The area where the IV entered my hand felt like a bee sting. When we arrived at the shower area, the glare of lights put Jean in a spotlight of sorts as she stood close to me. Her face was scarred by acne. Her thin red hair was pulled back in a tight bun, but wisps fell down and across her face. Occasionally, she brushed them away with the back of her hand, but to no avail. Despite the scarred face and messy hair, a pair of the kindest green eyes shone behind wire-rimmed glasses.

The shower became a balancing act for Jean, one that she handled beautifully. She held me around the waist with one hand and washed me with her other. Being rubbed down with a cool washcloth and feeling the water splashing down my spine took me back to happier days when my mother gave me a bath as a child. Then Jean washed my long dark hair like a hairdresser would, gently rubbing my scalp. I didn't want my shower to end.

Once it was over, Jean dressed me in a new gown and wrapped my hair in towels. After helping me back to bed, she spent her time off towel-drying my tresses. Some of my pain must have washed down the drain in the shower or worn off onto the fuzzy towels.

"Thank you," I said, my voice barely audible.

"Somebody on days should have given you a sponge bath. Anything else I can do?"

"No. You've done enough."

"Just want to help. I can definitely see you're hurting. I'll be back on the night shift, girlie."

After Jean left, I tried resting. Sleep still wouldn't come. The fever hung on tenaciously.

But Jean stood at my bedside every night, whispering, "You can beat this. God is on your side."

It took five more days for my fever to break. After it did, the doctors sent me home.

I didn't get to say goodbye to Jean. I tried contacting her later at the hospital, but they said she didn't work that floor anymore. I couldn't find her in the directory either. It would have been nice to thank her.

While convalescing at home, a friend sent me a book about angels. Leafing through it, I smiled. I knew how it felt to be visited by angels. They're like Jean. There's no need to wear corrective lenses to see them. Their wings rustle like tight-fitting polyester. And their shoes squeak. Just loudly enough so you'll remember you were in their presence.

~Jill Davis

Angel at My Bedside

Thy purpose firm is equal to the deed. Who does the best his circumstance allows, does well, acts nobly; angels could do no more.
~Edward Young

The subdued lights and muted voices frightened me. I could sense the tension and worry in the room. Something was wrong. Women had babies every day and I'd never heard of any of my friends being whisked away into a dark, isolated area filled with strange intimidating monitors.

I was three weeks past my due date, and although my labor was induced, I suspected the dull ache I'd been feeling in my lower back all day heralded my child's intent to finally enter the world. The dripping tube connected to my arm was simply speeding up the process. Hushed whispers, the worry on my husband Don's ashen face and his weak assurances that everything was all right only increased my anxiety.

Despite the epidural I'd been given, my discomfort grew. A roaring pressure reverberated in my head. I heard moaning, then screams of pain. As they grew louder, I realized they were coming from me.

A cool palm touched my feverish forehead and I glanced up to see gentle eyes behind a masked face. "I'm Debbie, your nurse. I know you're frightened and you're hurting, but we're taking good care of you. Trust us, okay?"

I nodded, then groaned as another cramp ripped through me. When it dissipated, I became aware of a doctor at the foot of my bed. He examined me while Debbie grasped my hand, positioning herself so she blocked him from my view. A tilt of my head, however, exposed his worried face.

"I want you to breathe with me," the nurse instructed, distracting me. "I understand it's difficult, but we need you relaxed and calm, so follow what I do." She proceeded to inhale and slowly exhale. I tried to imitate her, but all I could do was pant. "Focus" she crooned. "Close your eyes and count to ten with each breath."

I attempted to follow her example, but another agonizing contraction tore at me. My husband gripped my hand, urging me to squeeze as hard as I could. I heard voices emanating from a dark corner of the room. Doctors conferring. The grim, barely audible way they spoke terrified me. "Severe toxemia." "Danger of stroke." "High blood pressure." "Not rotating properly." "C-section."

Staff tiptoed in and out. The dim lights were finally turned off altogether, replaced by flashlights when my vital signs were checked. Eventually, even my husband was asked to leave. I began to cry and protest.

"Shh," Debbie soothed hypnotically. "He'll be in the waiting room, but I'll stay. I'm not going anywhere." Her voice had a mesmerizing effect on me, lulling me through my haze of agony.

As promised, she didn't leave my side, asking me questions about myself, showing genuine interest, and amusing me with anecdotes about her job. As she chattered, her eyes darted to the various monitors and machines. She illuminated my chart with the weak rays of her penlight to jot down the information she read.

I don't know how much time elapsed. Pain and fear mingled together. Every time I became too distressed or incoherent, Debbie managed to pacify me by stroking my hair, wiping my face with a cool cloth, murmuring quietly, or asking questions.

Doctors continued to enter and exit the room, conferring with each other out of my earshot, but their grave expressions were impossible to ignore. Finally, after what seemed like an eternity, one of them approached my bed, where I was balled up in a fetal position.

"We're going to take you into the delivery room, now," he announced. "You're fully dilated."

"My husband," I croaked, clamping on to Debbie's arm. "I told him I didn't want him in the delivery room, but now I do. Please, can you ask him to come?"

"He'll be there," she promised.

I was wheeled down a long hallway. Debbie walked briskly beside my gurney, continuously soothing me with soft-spoken words and reassuring smiles.

"You're coming in too!" I demanded rather than asked.

"Of course!" she grinned. "After I wash up and get a gown on."

"My husband?"

"He'll be right behind me."

After that, everything became a blur. I thrashed and cried as I was pushed through swinging doors, only relaxing when I recognized familiar eyes behind masks—both my husband's and my nurse's. Then suddenly my world went black.

I woke to the sounds of a baby's lusty cries. Turning my head weakly, I saw a small bundle in Don's arms.

"You have a beautiful, healthy son," someone told me, as my eyes closed again.

The next time I opened them, I was in another darkened room. I groaned and heard some movement at my right. From the dim glow of the hall lights, I could make out a human form sitting in a chair beside me.

"Don?" I called, through parched lips.

"It's me—Debbie," came the response. "We sent your hubby home. But I'm still here."

She stood and approached me, reaching for a small carafe of water. She poured some into a glass and raised my head to take a sip.

"I wanted to make sure you were okay," she told me, adjusting my pillow. "Drink this and try to sleep some more. You've had a rough time."

"My baby?"

"He's perfect," she assured me. "He weighed in at eight pounds ten ounces. You'll see him in the morning. Right now he's screaming down in the nursery with those strong lungs of his."

I drifted off again. Every time I awoke, it was to find that dedicated nurse right beside me, seeing to my every need.

Finally, sunlight streamed through the drawn blinds of the quiet room. I opened my eyes to see Don sitting in the chair Debbie had vacated, relief evident on his face.

"Welcome back," he whispered, wrapping his arms around me. "You had us all scared for a while, but you're going to be okay."

I stared at him, puzzled.

He explained that I had preeclampsia, and that I almost died. My obstetrician had missed the warning signs of toxemia. Luckily, both my baby and I were fine.

That afternoon, I walked a little and stopped at the nurse's station to ask where I could find Debbie.

"She left on vacation as soon as she was sure you'd recover," the head nurse told me. "She was terribly worried about you and changed her flight because she didn't want to leave you."

Stunned, I asked, "Why on earth would she do that?"

"That's Debbie," she replied.

Although I never saw that wonderful, dedicated nurse again, several weeks later, I called to thank her. Her voice on the phone was as caring and kind as I remembered, and I could almost see her shrug humbly when I babbled my thanks for her devotion and care.

Over the years, I've learned one universal truth. Nurses are angels at the bedside.

~Marya Morin

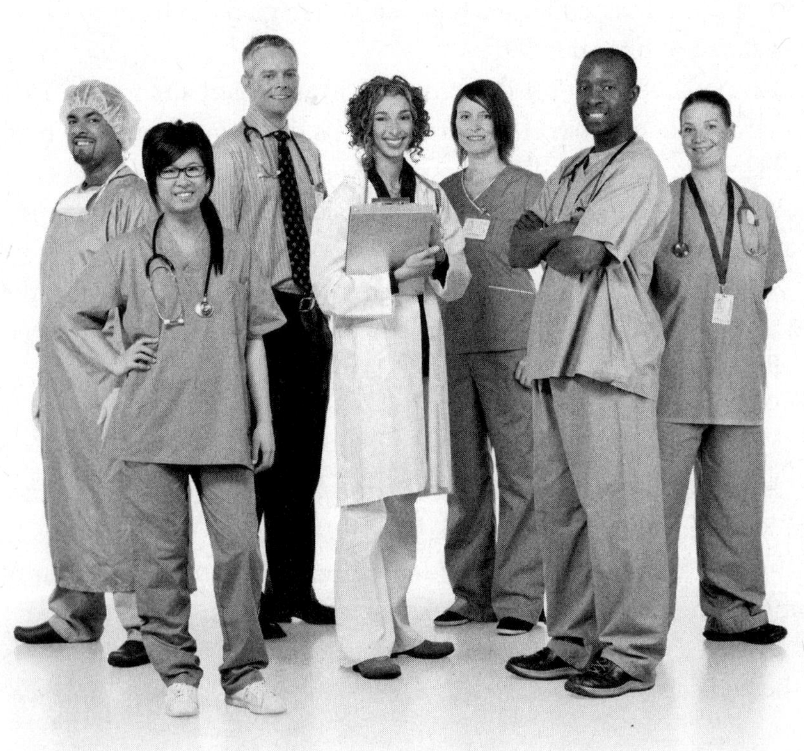

Inspiration for Nurses

A Matter of Perspective

Try to see things differently — it's the only way to get a clearer perspective on the world and on your life.

~Neal Shusterman

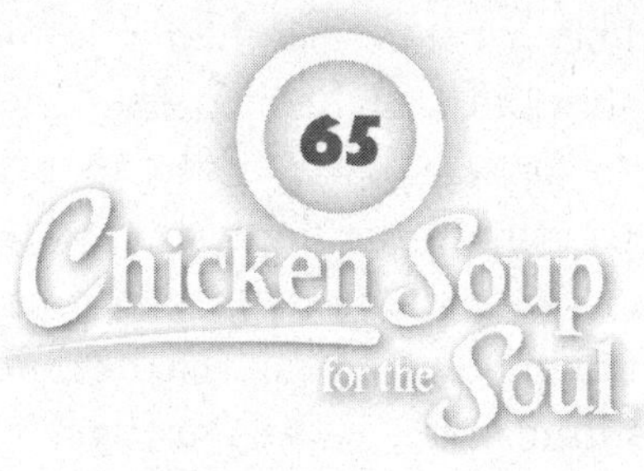

It's Not What You Lose

A thousand words will not leave so deep an impression as one deed.
~Henrik Ibsen

My husband, Jude, suffered his first heart attack when he was thirty-eight years old. He had been sailing on Lake Huron with our seven-year-old son, who miraculously followed my husband's instructions and brought the boat safely into harbour.

Jude changed his diet, began exercising regularly, and valiantly attempted to stop smoking. He purchased a filter for the cigarettes and then tried a pipe and then added a highly touted filter for the pipe, all to no avail. The tobacco and its additives had him in its grip.

There were two more heart operations—both of them bypasses. Then five years later, the dreaded but predictable diabetes, awaiting many heart patients, set in.

Panic gripped both of us as one doctor after another made the diagnosis that his left leg from below the knee down needed to be amputated.

The evening before the slated operation, I sat on the side of his hospital bed and held him in my arms as he cried. "I won't be able to live like this," he told me. "A walker. Crutches. A cane. Hobbling along behind you and the boys. Nothing to do but sit. Nowhere to go. I'm too young for this." He truly believed he no longer had a life worth living. I had never before seen him in such a state of absolute despair, so thoroughly and wretchedly defeated.

We sat facing the far side of the private room and hadn't noticed the nurse quietly pausing in the doorway. The tentative clearing of a throat alerted us to his presence. "If I may?" he spoke with gentle respect. "I couldn't help but overhear." He held up the stack of linen and hospital robes in his arms. "I was just coming in to stash these and... well, I heard... and..." He looked both abashed and determined. "I'm going to do something I've never done before. If I may?" he repeated.

And then, perhaps fearing that his courage would wane if he waited for our consent, which might or might not be given, he placed his bundle on a vacant chair and, taking one of the blue gowns, stepped into the bathroom. Moments later, the door opened. "It was a motorcycle accident," he said softly but clearly as he looked into Jude's swollen, startled eyes. "I was twenty-one."

There stood our nurse, his gown wrapped demurely just below his underwear line. His soft-soled shoes and sports socks defined in sharp contrast to the flesh color of his prosthetics. "Both legs," he said. "One above the knee. One below."

Jude sat, stunned, blinking back his tears.

"It's taken me a few years," the nurse continued shyly. "I'm twenty-six now. But while I healed my body and my mind, while I did session after session of therapy, I also went to school... maybe something I otherwise never would have done. Who knows? But as it was, I received a degree in nursing. I still play soccer—granted not as well as I would have in the Coast League where I played before, but I still play. I'm getting married next month and when I have kids, well..." He pointed to his prosthetic legs. "I guess what I've learned through all of this is that it's not what we lose, like in our cases our legs, but what we do with what we've still got that really decides the outcome of..." He paused to draw a heavy breath, "...the rest of our lives."

And at that, he turned back to the washroom, one leg of his bright red boxers showing below the unassuming blue hospital gown.

Jude slipped back against his pillow. “That young nurse…” He paused to shake his head. “After the operation, tomorrow, we’ll get started on our new future. I’m ready.”

~Robyn Gerland

A Shower of Gifts

Death may be the greatest of all human blessings.
~Socrates

Buzz. Buzz. Buzz. The rattle of my pager dancing across the bedside table brought me out of a deep sleep. It took a few seconds to figure out what woke me. Buzz. Buzz. Buzz.

"Rats," I muttered, and silenced the torture device. I grabbed my phone and left the bedroom before my husband woke. "Please God, not today," I whispered, and headed downstairs for my notepad and computer.

As an organ transplant coordinator, I frequently worked twenty-four-hour call shifts that started at 6:00 a.m. My shift had begun.

I loved my job helping families through the sudden death of a loved one by offering them the opportunity to save lives through organ and tissue donation. Most families viewed this as the only positive outcome of the worst day of their lives. I wanted to advocate for the thousands of people on the waiting list.

I just didn't want to do it that day.

My first grandchild was due and a baby shower was planned for that afternoon. I didn't mind working all day and night; I just wanted to go to the shower for a few hours.

Before I dialed the number on the pager screen I uttered a prayer. It was admittedly selfish. "Please God; let it be at a nearby hospital.

Or someone not close to being brain dead. Or maybe someone not medically suitable to donate."

A tired voice gave me the brief details of my assignment. I'd get the rest of the information from the ICU nurse. I hurriedly dressed and grabbed my equipment and the baby shower gift. Just in case.

While en route I spoke with the ICU nurse. The patient, Yvonne, was a forty-five-year-old woman with a ruptured blood vessel in her brain. She had been healthy until she complained of a headache and collapsed. The medical team had completed the first set of tests to determine brain death.

My heart sank. I would not be going to my daughter's baby shower. I cried as I called her. "I'm sorry, honey. I just got called out on a case and I don't think I'll make it to your shower." I heard her sniffling when we ended the call.

I wiped my eyes and gave myself a mental shake. It was time to focus on the needs of this family. After all, I was about to celebrate a birth; they faced a death. How could I complain?

The next twenty-four hours were a blur. I scoured all of Yvonne's medical records while the staff repeated the brain death tests. When she was officially pronounced brain dead, I met with the family. They were devastated. They had cried, prayed and begged for a miracle ever since she'd collapsed at home just twelve hours before. How could this happen to their lovely, healthy child, wife, sister?

I had no answers.

"Tell me about Yvonne," I said. The room was quiet for ten seconds and then one by one her grieving family shared how loving, sweet and kind she was. Her husband shared stories of her generosity.

"That's right," her brother said. "She would give you the shirt off her back."

"I am so sorry for your loss. From all the wonderful things you've told me, I'm sure I would have liked her. As you know, Yvonne was pronounced brain dead at 10:00, but because she is still on the ventilator and on certain medications, her heart is still beating. I am so sorry you did not receive the miracle you prayed for, but she has the opportunity to be the miracle for several people who desperately need an organ transplant." I paused so they could absorb the information.

"It's not often people die in this manner, but it's the only way a person can receive an organ, other than kidneys, from living donors."

Yvonne's parents looked at her husband, wiping their eyes. "What do you think? Did she want to be an organ donor?"

"I know she didn't put it on her license but we never really discussed it," he said.

I turned to Yvonne's brother. "Dan, you said she would give you the shirt off her back. If she knew she could save the lives of up to eight people, what do you think she would say?"

Four people answered in unison. "Yes."

"Can she really save that many lives?" Her husband's voice choked.

It was my turn to answer. "Yes."

It took almost twenty hours to make all the arrangements. Tests were needed to assess the health of each organ that was gifted. I needed to work with UNOS, the United Network for Organ Sharing, to identify the recipients, then arrange for the surgical teams to come recover those organs.

As I worked through the night my mind wandered to my family a few times. I thought about the baby shower, but of course didn't mention it to anyone as I plowed ahead with my tasks.

The organ recovery was underway and going well when a coworker arrived to relieve me. After reporting to her, I stumbled to the ICU waiting area to speak with the family. Although most families say goodbye to their loved ones and leave immediately after the consent is signed, this family vowed to stay until the donation process was completed.

They stood as one when I stepped into the room. I noticed they wore identical expressions of concern and I assured them. "All is well."

I folded into an empty chair. The adrenaline rush had worn off and I was suddenly exhausted. "My coworker Diane is here to relieve me. She knows you're waiting and she'll be up to speak with you after she finishes with Yvonne's care. Again, I am so sorry for your loss. You have a wonderful, kind family and it has been my pleasure to be with you through this journey."

When I stood and extended my hand to her family, I was engulfed in one powerful embrace after another. Her husband and parents thanked me. "You are so kind, Judy. God bless you," her mother said as she hugged me.

Dan, Yvonne's baby brother, spoke through tears. "Please tell your family how much we needed you today and how much you helped us. I know they must miss out on a lot of time with you since you're away for such long hours. Let them know we appreciate their sacrifice."

I was humbled and embarrassed by my earlier prayers and resentment. Although I couldn't attend the baby shower, the gifts given that night were better than any that my daughter had unwrapped. Yvonne's courageous family showered the gift of life onto six people.

~Judy Pencek

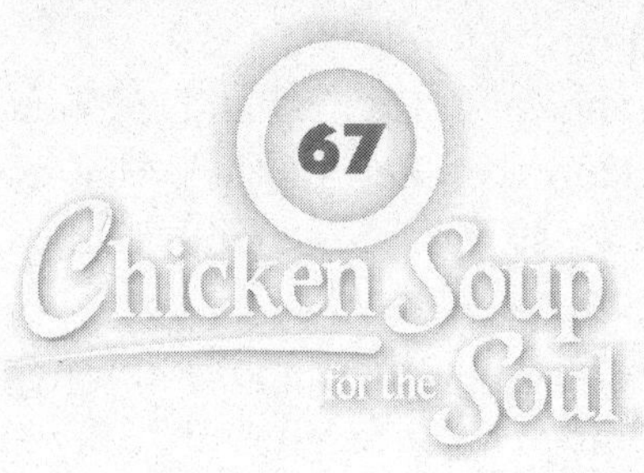

Things Aren't Always What They Seem

If you make listening and observation your occupation, you will gain much more than you can by talk.
~Robert Baden-Powell

I had several years of hospital work experience behind me when I made the switch to community-based home health care. I loved the idea of being one-on-one with my patients, and especially seeing them in their home environment. My assigned territory with my new agency took me to a neighborhood where many people would hesitate to go. My initial trepidation was quickly replaced by a sincere appreciation for the people who lived and persevered in this often dangerous and generally neglected neighborhood.

Mrs. Johnson was first on my list. As I drove up to her tiny clapboard house, I saw the curtain on the front door window immediately pulled aside. She watched me as I sat in the car, documenting my mileage and time and gathering the necessary paperwork and equipment. I saw the curtain continuously twitching back and forth, and thought to myself, "Another Nervous Nellie."

Some folks got genuinely agitated about having a stranger in their home and I anticipated wasting time on allaying her fears. But after Mrs. Johnson ushered me inside, and quickly locked and bolted the door, she sat on her sagging couch and smiled expectantly at me, her bright, intelligent eyes showing no sign of worry or fear.

I proceeded with my detailed assessment, ticking off a long list of health-related questions. We spoke at length about her medical history and I explained the primary reason for my visit. There were concerns about her blood pressure and uncontrolled diabetes after a recent hospitalization, and her physician wanted home health to work with her to get both of these under better control. I quickly checked her vital signs, reviewed her medications, and began to discuss my goals for her plan of care.

"Is there anything else going on that I need to know about?" I asked her at last.

"Well" she said hesitantly, "I don't sleep well at night."

"Okay," I replied, thinking this was pretty minor and not unusual with elderly people. "We'll see how that goes over time," I said, making a notation on my form.

I finished my paperwork and took my leave. Mrs. Johnson showed the same haste and agitation she had on my arrival.

This became her usual pattern. I talked about diabetes and hypertension. Mrs. Johnson listened quietly, followed my instructions, but continued to make reference to her ongoing inability to sleep. She was still waiting nervously at the door when I arrived, and watched constantly after I left until I pulled away from the curb. After several weeks, she showed marked improvement in her blood pressure and blood sugar readings. I felt pleased with my ability to help her achieve these established goals and knew our visits together would soon come to an end. I felt, since our primary goals had been achieved, we should address her persistent sleep issues.

"So, why don't we talk a little bit more about your sleep problems?" I finally asked her, thinking a call to her primary physician might be in order. "Maybe your doctor would want you to have a sleeping pill."

After some hesitation she said, "Oh, it's not like that. I don't need a sleeping pill."

"Why don't you tell me what you think the problem is? Obviously this is something that has been bothering you for a while."

Taking a deep breath, Mrs. Johnson began. "Oh honey, I am so worried about you when you come to see me early in the morning like this. See that empty lot behind my house?"

Now I was really confused, but I said that I did, wondering how this had anything to do with anything.

"Every night when the sun goes down," she continued, "those drug dealers come out and hang around the back of the house there. Now, my bedroom is in the back of the house, and there's no way I'm sleeping in there, what with all the shooting, and fighting, and bullets whizzing by. No sir! This old house is nothing but boards and I might get shot right there in my bed! So I come out here and sleep on this old couch."

I looked at the sagging couch in dismay, visualizing this precious lady trying to get comfortable on that lumpy old couch with visible springs poking through. And the walls were, in fact, nothing but the inside of the outside clapboards, and I could see daylight between most of them. But she wasn't done yet, and her next words dismayed me.

"I am so afraid for you when you come here in the morning. Sometimes those drug dealers are still out there, and I'm scared to death somebody will shoot you. I just don't have a moment's peace until you are safely inside this door. And you know I don't see that well, so when you leave, I wait to hear your car pull away; then I know you made it back to your car and are safely on your way."

As I looked into the face of this little lady who had endured so much, I was overwhelmed and ashamed. I had made judgments about her, decided what was best for her, and established an agenda that never once included issues important to her. And all the while, her concern was only for me.

Obviously, I could not change how or where she lived or eliminate the criminal element in her neighborhood. I realized, though, that a few modifications in my behavior could make a big difference in reducing her stress and worry.

For the remainder of the time that I saw her, I did not do paperwork in my car. I went into her house promptly and left the same way. It gave her peace of mind and gave me the satisfaction of knowing I made her day a little easier.

Now, many years after that eye-opening experience, I know I am a better nurse for having known Mrs. Johnson. It's great to have goals and a plan, but real nursing care takes your patient's needs and feelings into account first. I have learned to be a better listener, to judge less, and to adapt my goals based on my patient's priorities rather than my own.

Most importantly, I have come to realize that things aren't always what they seem. And sometimes, that's a positive learning experience for everyone.

~Sharon Stoika-Smay

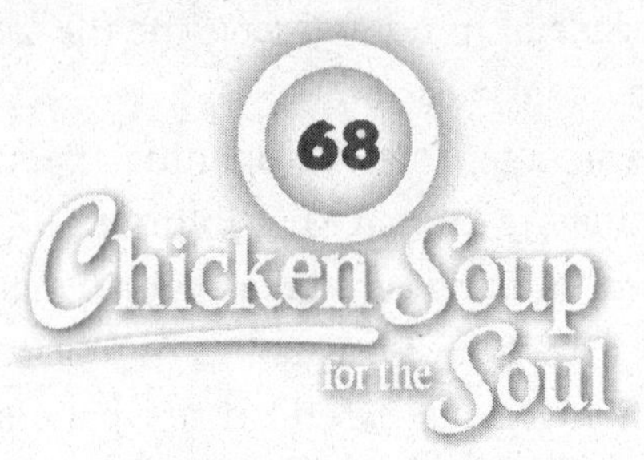

Who's Paying Attention?

Three things cannot be long hidden: the sun, the moon, and the truth.
~Buddha

I was the clinical instructor for a community college's Associate Degree Nursing program and my students were completing their last term on a large medical unit. Their objectives were to function independently, knowing when to ask for help while practicing their critical thinking and organizational skills.

Amy was assigned to care for Ella, a 100-year-old skilled–nursing home resident who was hospitalized for recurrent wound infections. Ella had many dressing changes, IVPB antibiotics, a GT feeding, and numerous medications. Amy spent long hours at Ella's bedside and was appropriately independent. My role was to stand at the opposite side of the bed, supervising, offering encouragement, and supporting Amy as needed.

Ella's level of consciousness varied. She did not answer questions appropriately, was not oriented to time or place, and was frequently combative. She was almost always yelling, singing, or calling for people who weren't there. Most of the time her eyes were closed, but she did seem to take comfort from reassurances and gentle touch.

At the end of the last day of the clinical assignment, Amy was completing her care while Ella jabbered on, with me standing by as usual. When she was just about finished with the laborious process, Amy asked me a question.

Ella interrupted her ranting, stopped thrashing, opened her eyes, looked at Amy, and yelled, "What the hell are you asking her for? She hasn't done anything all week! All she does is stand there!"

Amy and I both roared with laughter and told Ella we agreed with her.

I am sure Ella's comment did more for Amy's confidence that day than any evaluation I could have given her.

~Mary Lynn Harrison

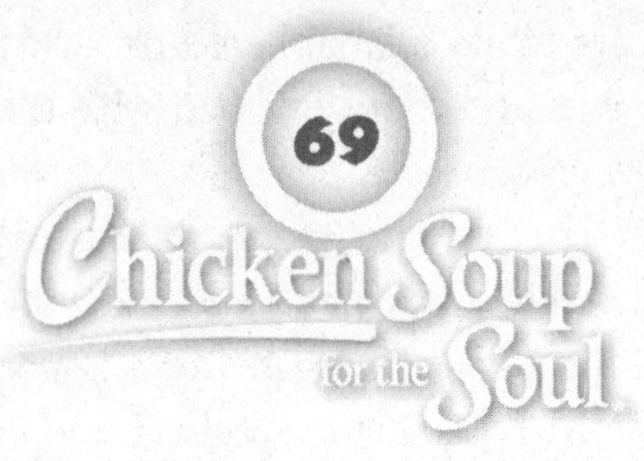

A Nurse Named Michael

Those who learn to know death, rather than to fear and fight it, become our teachers about life.
~Elisabeth Kübler-Ross

Larry had been complaining about a pain in his hip for quite some time. Instead of getting better, it worsened. Normally he avoided doctors, but the pain became unbearable and he had no choice but to make an appointment with our family physician.

When X-rays did not reveal the cause of the pain, he was referred to an orthopedic specialist who ordered an MRI. My worst fears were confirmed. Larry had prostate cancer that had metastasized to his bones.

The oncologist was honest and forthright in responding to our questions. Larry was much better at accepting the answers than I. The cancer was aggressive and terminal, but he could live up to three years by actively treating it.

After weighing the pros and cons of cancer therapy, we took the doctor's advice. Larry began a combination of chemotherapy and radiation treatments immediately. There was never a question in my mind. I was adamant; we were going to fight this with any and all available means.

As expected, the treatments made Larry very weak and nauseated. And the cancer continued to spread. The doctor told us that another round of chemo might be helpful. Although Larry was hesitant, I, in my selfish need to keep him with me as long as possible, stubbornly turned a blind eye to the dreaded side effects. I persuaded him to continue with additional rounds of chemo and other treatments until nearly every option was exhausted. And the cancer continued to spread.

On our last visit the oncologist said, "Well, Larry, there is one more option. I think I can get you approved for a clinical trial with a new cancer-fighting drug. How would you feel about that?"

I squealed ecstatically, "Oh yes, of course! Anything. We'll try anything!"

My mouth fell open when I heard Larry sob. "I can't do this anymore. I am so sorry, but I just can't."

I couldn't believe what he was saying. How could he just give up and die? I felt betrayed and angry.

Since Larry, not I, was his patient, the doctor wasn't about to force him do something simply because his wife insisted. As we left for home, I convinced myself that I could change his mind with a little pleading.

Larry worsened quickly. A few days later, unable to keep food down, he was admitted to the hospital. Since there were no available rooms on oncology, he was given a bed on the post-operative floor, where patients were recovering from surgeries.

Although nurses came in and out of the room, I felt like Larry was mostly ignored because they had no idea what to do for him. They were used to dealing with post-op rather than terminal patients.

I felt neglected, as if nobody cared. We were alone in this huge hospital and all I could do was pray, so I did—a simple appeal for comfort and guidance.

Soon after I uttered my prayer, a tall young man in dark blue scrubs walked into the room. He introduced himself as Michael, our nurse for the evening shift.

I thought, "Just when I thought things couldn't get worse, they've sent in a mere child to care for my husband." I was certain he would take one look at this pathetic sick man and walk out the door just like the other nurses.

Instead, Michael grabbed a chair and scooted it over to my husband's bedside. Sitting, he leaned in close. "How are you feeling, Larry?"

"I'm sorry, but I just want to give up and go home."

He was so young, yet the nurse spoke with the wisdom of someone much older. "I know you're tired, Larry. These treatments are brutal. If you decide to discontinue them, you shouldn't feel as though you're a failure. The life you've lived up to this point is what's important, and that's what your family and friends will remember about you. They don't want you to have to be sick every day. They'd rather spend quality time with you."

He turned to make sure I was listening before continuing. "My grandpa died a few months ago from cancer. The very best decision we made was to get hospice involved so he could live his final days in comfort. Like you, he didn't want additional therapy just to prolong his life for a short time, so we respected his wishes. I'll never forget my grandpa and all he taught me."

He then turned toward me. "I really hope you will consider giving hospice a call. They are wonderful."

Knowing this young man had experienced what my kids and grandchildren were going through touched me to the core. Until then, no one had suggested hospice. Perhaps they sensed, correctly, that I'd resist. This young nurse, however, opened my eyes, making me finally concede that this was Larry's life, not mine; the choice was his to make.

The following morning, as Larry was being discharged, Michael appeared again. I watched as he gently and respectfully helped Larry dress and get into the wheelchair. He grabbed warm blankets, tucking one around his shoulders and another over his legs. When we got to the car, he carefully helped Larry into the passenger seat before saying, "Wait a moment; I'll be right back." He returned with two pillows, one he expertly placed behind Larry's back, and the other behind his legs. He wished us luck as he waved goodbye.

For the first time in my life, I realized that nursing was as much about communication as about physical care. Because of Michael, we had two precious, quality-filled months with Larry before he peacefully left us.

Nurses heal by offering care… and sometimes by modifying it.

~Connie Kaseweter Pullen

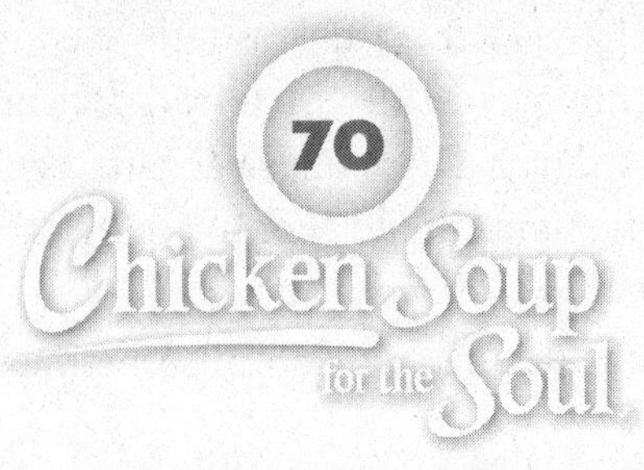

What a Nurse Sees

A warm smile is the universal language of kindness.
~William Arthur Ward

I never really understood the fear of hospitals. Growing up I heard people say, "Hospitals are creepy." Or, "I hate hospitals... all those sick people. Yuck."

But for me, I grew up in a hospital. My mom was a registered nurse for thirty-five years at Northgate, a small hospital wedged between a movie theater and a Red Robin. Hardly intimidating.

I was always walking the halls of that hospital for one reason or another. We would swing by to pick up her paycheck or run in so she could rework some schedule changes. As a busy nursing supervisor, she'd sometimes be called into work last minute. Sitters were hard to find on short notice, so I'd have to tag along with her. My sitter was often an empty hospital room.

I'd pretend I was in a hotel. Mom brought me a plastic pitcher of water with a little Dixie cup. We'd walk down to the cafeteria and get candy from the vending machine. But best of all, she'd bring me a warm blanket and wrap me up as I fell asleep.

Randomly, a smiling nurse would pop into the room to check on me. They'd shoot me a big smile and a wave, then continue on with their rounds.

I was never scared. Actually it was just the opposite. I felt so safe and cozy. Sometimes I wished we could live there. The nurses were the most loving, kind, and smiley people I'd ever met. Right behind my mom, of course.

All my younger years I'd been witness to the comforts of Mom's work. I saw how nurses made it their life's work to care for others. Not just care, but give all they had to save lives and heal the very sickest people.

But as I grew into a teenager, my overnights at the hospital ended. My experiences with warm blankets and kind-hearted nurses were replaced by make-up and boys. My own confusion and "creepy" thoughts of the hospital started to fester. Blood, guts, yuck.

One day my mom told me a story about a man in a motorcycle accident. "You could grab his nose and move it from one side of his face to the other. His whole face had been fractured."

"Mom! Gross! Why? Why do you do this job?"

She said, "Honey, nurses don't see what you see. You see broken bones, blood and guts. We… we see someone who needs our help. And that's all we see."

I will never forget that comment. "We see someone who needs our help. And that's all we see."

What an amazing life lesson. Wouldn't it be a beautiful world if we all saw what a nurse sees? What if we didn't see the brokenness of a human? What if we didn't see the gory blood and guts? What if we just saw a human being who needed our help?

Oh what a world it would be, if we could all just see what a nurse sees.

~Diana Lynn

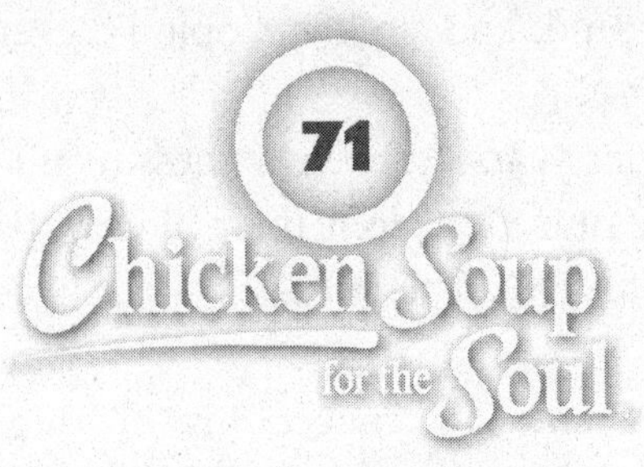

Not So Alone After All

This is the message of Christmas: We are never alone.
~Taylor Caldwell

Christmas in Tucson. I suppose that sounds exotic. Or at least warm. But it didn't feel like that to me.

I had moved from the Midwest to Arizona in January and quickly found a job as a nurse in one of the area hospitals. I had worked previously on a cardiac floor, so I was hired for the evening shift on a cardiac telemetry wing. I loved the fast pace, learning more about heart arrhythmias, and counseling patients and families on the treatments.

As one of the most recent hires, I worked most holidays. I knew I didn't have a prayer of getting Christmas off. All the other nurses had seniority. My boyfriend, a college student at the University of Arizona, flew home for his Christmas break. The nurse I moved to Tucson with somehow finagled the holiday off, so she was gone, too.

I didn't realize how hard my first Christmas away from home would be.

"I'll be fine." I told myself. I called home a few times, but hearing the voices and all the plans for the holiday made me long to be there on Christmas morning. By the time Christmas Eve came, my twenty-three-year-old heart was hurting. I was a lonely Midwest girl in the middle of the Southwestern desert.

After my Christmas Eve shift, I attended church at midnight. The familiar songs and prayers began to lift my mood. At the end of the service, I slowly made my way to the exit. As I passed the glowing candlelight and poinsettias, I came face to face with the pastor. I offered my hand and choked out, "Merry Christmas," while fighting off tears.

He tipped his head to one side and looked into my eyes. I knew he wanted to ask me what was wrong. I knew if he did, my fragile façade of Christmas cheer would crack and collapse into pieces. I hurried past him after mumbling something, and promptly burst into tears in the car.

Christmas day arrived. I made breakfast, and as I ate I gave myself a pep talk. "You already cried. Now you have to calm down. None of the patients want to be in the hospital for Christmas either." It was my job to be a cheerful face for everyone I'd see at the hospital. I made my phone call home, and after wishing them all a happy celebration, I was off to work.

I took report from the day nurse while silently wishing I was going home with her to a festive holiday dinner. Most of the patients had gone home for the holiday; maybe it would be a quiet night. I took a big breath, grabbed the medicine cart and started my rounds.

With a smile plastered on my face, I entered the first room., "Merry Chri…" I began to say, but the man in the first bed was up and shaking my hand.

"Merry Christmas! Have some of the cookies my family brought." He introduced me and they each thanked me for working on Christmas.

Before I knew it, I was nodding happily, shaking hands and accepting cookies. The mood in the room was so joyful, I couldn't be sad. "It's my pleasure," I responded, now with a real smile.

The man in the next bed chimed in. "We saved you some treats; I wouldn't let the day nurses eat it all," he said with pride as he offered me some fudge and fruitcake. He and his wife radiated joy too, in spite of having to spend this day in the hospital.

With each patient and family member I met, I could feel my heart healing. We were all a part of the "Christmas in the Hospital Club."

Finishing up my rounds, I entered the last room. The first bed was empty. In the next bed was a man in his thirties, which is young for a cardiac floor. I had taken care of him during the week. I saw he was alone in the dark, dozing on and off in front of a muted flickering television screen.

We exchanged a few pleasantries, but I could see he was feeling down. He told me that his family had come to visit earlier in the day. I knew just how he was feeling. He wasn't hundreds of miles away from his family, but he might as well have been.

I'm not sure how I thought of it. "Do you play poker?"

"I sure do," he said with a shy smile.

I found an old deck of cards at the nurse's station, and between caring for my other patients I ducked into his room to play five-card draw. Instead of poker chips, we played for paperclips. I could only stay for a hand or two, but every time I came in, he'd have the cards dealt, smiling and ready to play. I can't remember who won, but I do remember it was a lot of fun.

The end of my shift came. All the family members had left hours ago. Most of the patients were sleeping. The night shift nurses trickled in with stories of their celebrations and I actually enjoyed listening to them.

That Christmas day, I was the nurse, but my patients were the real healers.

~Ceil Ryan

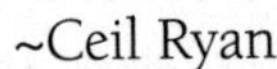

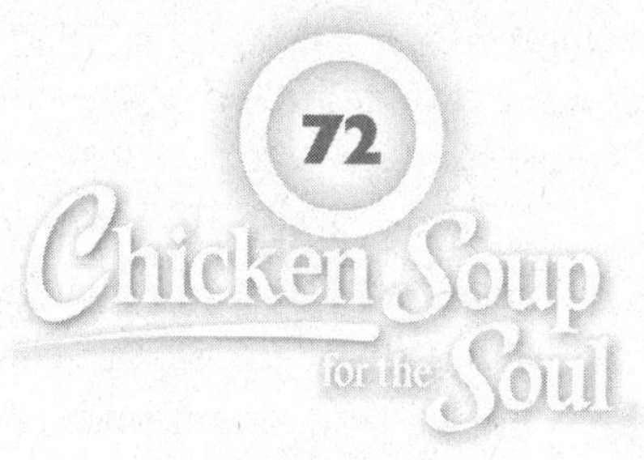

The Secret of Happiness

Happiness is not something ready made. It comes from your own actions.
~Dalai Lama

I wiped the sweat from my brow after moving my son into college and pulled the worn paper from my pocket. I reread the note given to me by my patient many years before and smiled. I'd feared this day would never come.

My son had many learning disabilities and by the second grade was still unable to read. I knew he was smart and I kept telling him that one day he would "read like a champ," but the truth was that some days I barely believed it myself. It was on one of those days that I walked into work at the Open Heart Surgery Intensive Care Unit and saw that Mr. Goodman had been readmitted.

I had known him for several years because he was a frequent patient in our ICU. Originally, he had contracted an infection in his heart valve that required a valve replacement, and he had been in and out of the hospital since. We had come to know him well and grew to love both him and his wife.

On this particular evening, as I trudged into the ICU, my heart was filled with a panic that even my son's sweet blue eyes had been able to see. His learning disabilities seemed insurmountable. When I saw Mr. Goodman on my list, I was both happy to see him and sad he was back. As his condition deteriorated, the success of our interventions was declining.

Although Mr. Goodman became sicker and sicker, his spirits and smile never waned. I looked at his progressive diagnosis and walked into his room. When I put my stethoscope to his chest, his lungs sounded full of fluid, but he smiled and said, "I'm here for another tune-up."

"I'll make certain we change the oil and fix the radiator then," I said, smiling back at him as I left the room. His wife soon came in and I heard them laughing. I have a PhD in worry and on this particular night I was overcome with worry for my son. I was drawn back into this room filled with laugher. "Mr. Goodman," I said, "you must know the secret of happiness because you are always smiling."

"I do," he replied. "Bring me a piece of paper and I will write it down for you."

Obediently, I brought him the paper. He proceeded to write and then handed me the note. It read: "The Secret of Happiness is not getting what you want, but wanting what you get." As I stared at his message, I was overwhelmed with the message it held for me. I felt tears well up as I realized that I'd only been concerned with getting what I wanted, instead of being thankful for what I had been given. He'd seen, on this night, that I needed his special wisdom. I took his hand. "Thank you."

As soon as I began to follow Mr. Goodman's secret of happiness, my fears and tears fell away like leaves on an autumn tree. Once I saw my son as the treasure he was, I lost my worry that he would never read. If he never read I would be grateful for his beautiful smile, the joy he found in everything he did, his contagious laugh and kind heart.

I gave Mr. Goodman his medications and changed his dressings, but he changed my perspective. From his note I learned that worrying about my son overcoming his disabilities only led to frustration for him and me. Acceptance of the gift life had given me led to peace.

Mr. Goodman surely didn't ask for the life he was given, and indeed it was not an easy one. Although he was not getting what he wanted, he wanted what he got and used that life to bring joy and laughter to the people around him. And on one dark night he brought wisdom to a weary, worrying nurse, who gratefully saved his note for a decade and a half. And, as it turned out, over time my son not only learned to read, but excelled at school.

~Alisa Edwards Smith

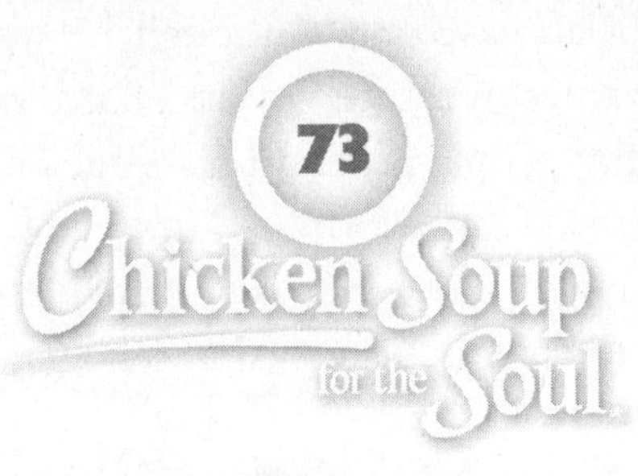

More Information

Next to a good soul-stirring prayer is a good laugh.
~Samuel Mutchmore

While manning the Telephone Care Unit at the psychiatric hospital where I worked, I received a call one evening from a man who identified himself as the manager of a chain restaurant across the street. I was extremely busy and there were several callers on hold awaiting my attention. He explained to me that one of our patients was at his restaurant.

"What do you mean you have one of our patients at your restaurant?" I asked.

"He is at the salad bar," the manager replied.

I was very annoyed at this point, because people sometimes stereotyped psychiatric patients. "Just because there is a man at your salad bar does not mean he is one of our patients," I responded hastily.

"He's naked."

"I'll send security to pick him up."

Sometimes you just need more information....

~C.J. Hopkins

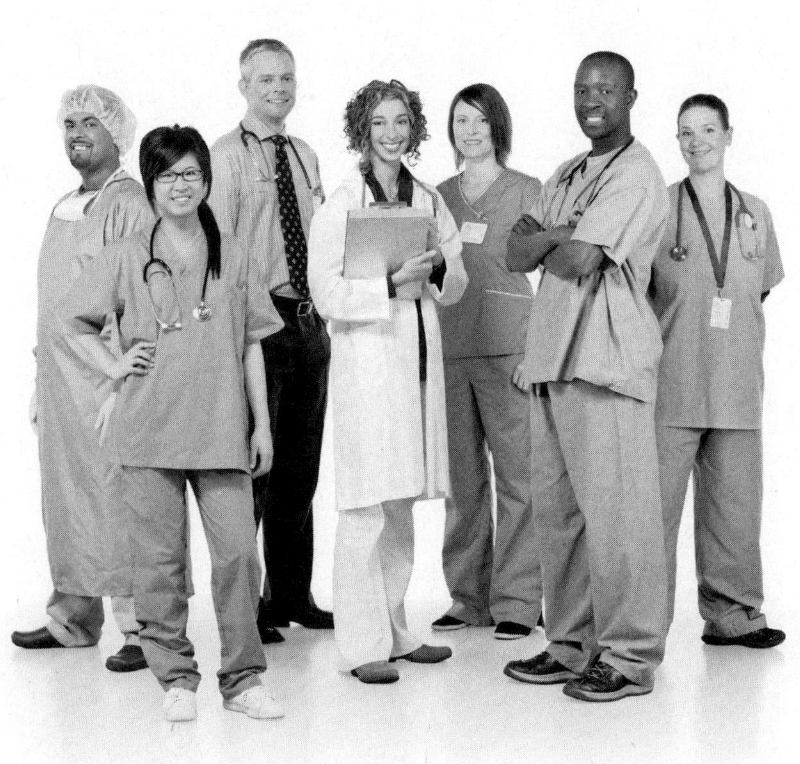

Inspiration for Nurses

Beyond the Call of Duty

The simple act of caring is heroic.

~Edward Albert

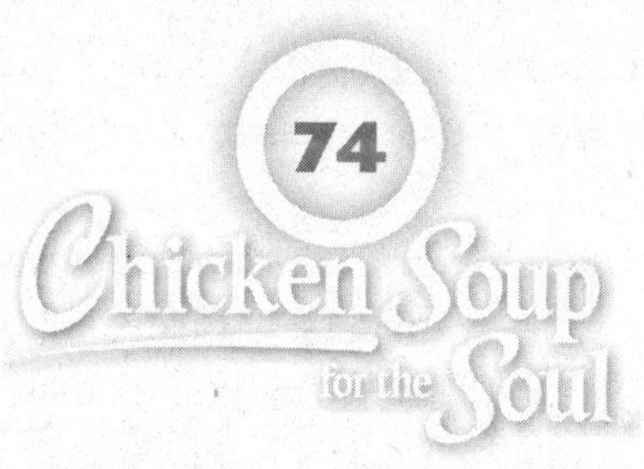

Merry Christmas Mr. J

It is one of the beautiful compensations of this life that no one can sincerely try to help another without helping himself.
~Charles Dudley

He was a proud war veteran, this man who changed my life. He lived alone in a tiny apartment and had no family left alive. He was fiercely independent, and now he was dying.

I was a fledgling hospice home health nurse working in a poor community that was fast becoming a ghost town, falling victim like so many others to the loss of once thriving industry. My husband had recently lost his job and we had a new home and mortgage. I was now the sole breadwinner and low on the pay scale. Christmas was coming. I was deeply depressed.

Mr. J came into my life uneventfully, another patient living in gang territory. I was used to the area and knew the necessary safety precautions. We were to visit early in the day and let the patient know when to expect us. We wore standard colors, easy to identify as "the nurse." We moved in and out of the homes quickly and left the area if there was any sign of trouble. I knew the rules and planned my day accordingly. Mr. J was my second visit of the day.

When I arrived I had that feeling of anticipation that only a home health nurse can know, the increasing adrenaline as you knock at the door wondering what you will find within. I knew only that he lived alone, was dying of cancer, and was discharged from the hospital the day before. Thoughts raced through my head. Did he know his prognosis? What kinds of problems was he having? Was he ready for hospice?

Mr. J opened the door, greeted me with a warm smile, and welcomed me in. The room was sparsely furnished but neat as a pin.

As we talked I learned that he had never married and had no one close, other than a few friends in the neighborhood. They took him to appointments and to the store. He was able to buy a few groceries with food stamps.

I noticed that the TV was on but had no picture. He saw me looking at it and got up to turn it off, telling me, "I listen to it; I don't need to see it anyway."

I asked about his sleeping arrangements and he pointed to the bedroom. I noticed he had no sheets, just a bare mattress with a blanket on top, stretched taut with nary a wrinkle, and tucked in tightly at the bottom. His corners were neater than any I had ever folded, perhaps from his military training. There was no sign of laundry anywhere, no chests or boxes, no hamper, nothing but a bed and a small closet. I peeked inside to see only a few pieces of tattered clothing on hangers.

As we turned toward the kitchen, I noted his clothes were so threadbare I could practically see through them.

I looked around with dawning awareness that this man had only a few items to his name. He had worked all his life but somehow ended up here, unable to afford any of the things that we think are so important to happiness. He was overwhelmingly poor, yet he was happy and kept his tiny apartment and his ragged clothes clean and neat as though he had a palace and the fine robes of a king.

He wanted nothing and denied any need for assistance or services. He was doing well the way things were, thank you very much, and would only allow the nurse to visit a few times to make his doctor happy. Nothing more. He knew he was dying, and that was okay with him for it was in God's hands and God had never failed him yet.

I cried that night. I felt so guilty for worrying about money and Christmas presents when in reality I had so much to be thankful for.

At the next visit I took him some sheets and a few pieces of clothing from my husband's closet. I lied, casually telling him that we had things in the office that people had given us for anyone who might be able to use them. If he took them that would really help us out since there was not much room in the office for storage. He agreed that would be just fine.

I wanted to do something for him for Christmas. I knew he would not want anyone to fuss over him. I thought of him all alone, listening to the TV, looking out at the snow, and it gave me an idea. My husband and I had combined our furniture when we married, and I still had the small TV from my apartment. It wasn't much, but it had a picture and Mr. J's did not. I decided that he should at least have a TV to watch at Christmas.

On Christmas Eve it was snowing heavily. We were headed to the annual family gathering, but I told my husband I needed him to do a favor for me before we went. We drove the dark winding road through the snow to where Mr. J lived. I was so excited, thinking that this was what it must be like to be Santa. I was concerned about going to the rough neighborhood after dark, but I knew that I had to do this.

When we got to the apartment complex, I had my husband take the TV to the door to give to Mr. J while I stayed hidden in the car. He had recently grown his beard and I had him wear a red Santa hat for the job.

When Mr. J opened the door, my husband said, "Merry Christmas! I heard you could use a TV!" He took it in, placed it on a table, turned and left.

We went on to the party, filled with happiness.

Mr. J died a few weeks later. We never spoke about the TV, but I saw it in the living room during my last few visits. I hope he watched something wonderful on Christmas Eve.

I like to think this one last gift for him made his last Christmas on earth as happy as he made mine.

~Carol Gaido-Schmidt

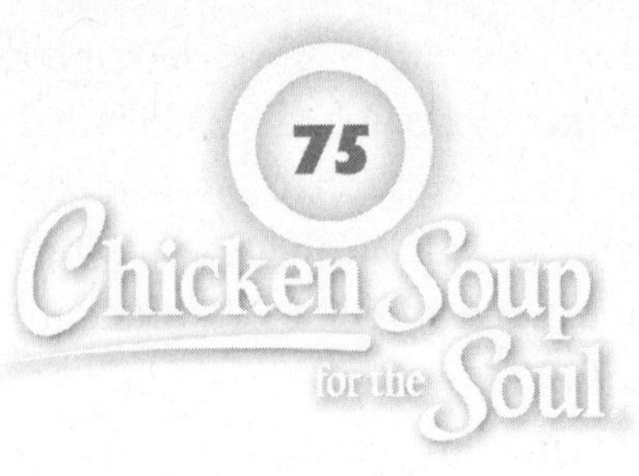

A Great Life If You Don't Weaken

Courage and perseverance have a magical talisman, before which difficulties disappear and obstacles vanish into air.
~John Quincy Adams

"I can't do this," I told my husband. "I don't remember a word they told us about it." Staring at the heparin solution and the hypodermic needle on the table and then looking at the Broviac-Hickman catheter coiled and taped in place against my daughter's side, I was numb.

I waved the written directions at my husband, who stammered, "My mind is too foggy to read those directions. I can't remember what they said about not getting air bubbles in the line."

Our daughter Kim mumbled, "Well, I can't do it and you can't do it; call Nadine."

Nadine was our neighbor who had worked at the local hospital, and then the school until retirement. Now she did private duty nursing. She was highly respected in the community and loved by children, including our daughter. To us, she was a good neighbor who was always saying, "It's a great life if you don't weaken." We didn't know why she said that, nor did we realize that someday we would find out.

During the week before we left the hospital, the chemotherapy nurses had given us directions on how to care for the Broviac-Hickman catheter when we got home. We knew we had to flush it three times daily with heparin solution to prevent blood clogging the line, and we also knew we had to flick the tubing to rid it of air bubbles. As we watched the competent nurses care for the catheter in the hospital and listened to what they said, the procedure seemed easy enough, and the three of us were confident we could at least do that during this time in our lives when everything seemed out of control.

Now we had just gotten home after a sixty-five-mile drive from the hospital in pouring rain with a nauseated daughter. As we entered our cold empty house, we suddenly realized it was time to flush the catheter. But all we felt like doing was crashing into bed exhausted. All our confidence had disappeared.

My husband turned on the heat and I looked toward Nadine's house. Although it was nearing midnight, her light was still on. I dialed her number and asked if she could come help us.

"I'll be right there." Within minutes, she came in our back door carrying a plate of homemade fried apple pies, Kim's favorite. She sat the plate on the table and headed toward the kitchen. "Mind if I put on a pot of hot coffee?" she asked. "That is, if the smell won't bother our girl. While I fix it, you can tell me what you need."

"Oh, the pies smell yummy, and I think I could eat one," Kim said. "The coffee smell isn't bothering me."

By the time we shared our need, Nadine had placed four cups of hot coffee on the table with four plates of fried apple pies. As the warm food coursed through our bodies and our house warmed, Nadine began preparing to flush the catheter as she chatted. "Now, let me share a little secret with you that I've learned in thirty years of nursing, on how to be sure there are no air bubbles." Before we knew it, the catheter was flushed, she had left, and we collapsed on our beds in exhaustion.

The next morning arrived and it was time to flush the catheter for the first time that day. I feared that task, and so did my husband. "Nadine said to call her anytime if I needed anything, so I'll just call her back." When I called again, she said she'd be glad to come over.

The minute she walked in, she started talking. "I've just had the most wonderful idea. I've been thinking of your hardworking family. Dad, you take care of your family, your yard, and your job. Mom, you are such an outstanding teacher as well as wife and mother. And dear Kim, you are so good in academics and work hard in all you do. I've decided since the catheter has to be flushed three times a day and there are three of you, you can all help me out. You know, a nurse also has to be a teacher to her patients, and last night I taught you a procedure. I am going to let Dad re-teach me what I taught him last night, as he does the first flush of the day. Then Mom, I want you to re-teach me the procedure on the second flush of the day. On the last flush, our sweet Kim can re-teach me what I taught you last night. Even old nurses need to brush up on their skills, and you'll be helping me see whether I'm a good teacher or not. After all, it's a great life if you don't weaken."

What a wise nurse. What a great teacher. By the end of the day, all three of us had flushed the catheter without air bubbles or problems, and our confidence had returned. We also understood, "It's a great life if you don't weaken."

~Helen Wilder

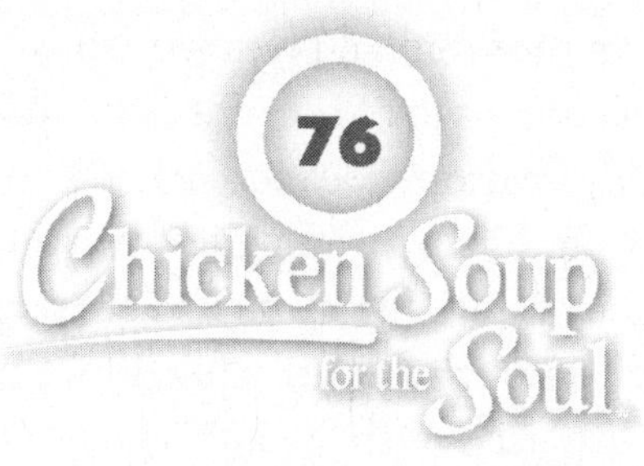

Caring Through Tragedy

Pain is the deepest thing we have in our nature, and union through pain and suffering has always seemed more real and holy than any other.
~Arthur Hallam

On a Sunday afternoon, a catastrophic car accident sent a thirty-two-week pregnant patient to our hospital in critical condition. The emergency department activated the OB emergent delivery team and the baby was delivered by emergency C-section. But he didn't survive. The Labor and Delivery nursing team was dismissed after the delivery of the infant, but they chose to stay.

"We'll complete the grief care for the baby and offer support to the grandmother who was in the car and is still in the Emergency Department."

The L&D nursing team took the baby to their L&D Bereavement room and began the customary bereavement care. They created hand and foot castings, made footprint cards, cut and packaged a lock of hair, bathed the baby, and dressed him in a smocked gown donated by a local church group. Recognizing that it would likely be several days before this mother could see or hold her baby, they called a local photographer to take professional photos of him.

Then the nurses went to the ED to check on the grandmother and to inform her of her grandson's location. After learning she would be in the ED several more hours awaiting test results, they brought the baby to her cradled in a soft blue blanket. The weeping grandmother asked, "Can one of you stay with me while I love my grandson?"

The nurse gently placed the baby in his grandmother's arms. "He's perfect," she said. After cuddling him and kissing him, she went on to express more feelings of hopelessness.

"I lost my cell phone in the accident, and can't remember any family numbers from back home. And I don't know if my three small dogs in the car survived."

The L&D nurse called the police department near the accident site to inquire about the cell phone and the dogs.

"They haven't found your cell phone, but your three dogs are safe and sound at the police station."

That evening, after she was discharged from the ED, the grandmother came to L&D to be with the baby again. The night staff noticed she was in paper scrubs.

The grandma shrugged. "My clothes were cut off. My suitcase was in the car. I don't have any of my clothes or underclothes."

The night shift team immediately went to work, pooling their money and rearranging assignments so someone could leave and go to the twenty-four-hour Walmart.

A few hours later, they reappeared and handed the grandma a shopping bag overflowing with clothes, undergarments, and toiletries. All she could do was weep and promise to pay them back as soon as she found her wallet.

"No need," the staff said through their own tears. "This is our gift to you."

The following day, the prognosis for the mother was very grim. The L&D nursing staff coordinated with the mother's ICU nurse to bring the infant to her so photographs could be taken for a lasting memory.

A few days later, the grandmother's friend arrived to be her support and help arrange a memorial service to honor the life of her grandson. The L&D nursing staff, chaplains and social workers assisted in coordinating a lovely service in the hospital chapel. The nurses rearranged their schedules, and when the grandmother walked into a chapel, a dozen nurses… new friends… greeted her.

I know this is a very difficult story to read, but I felt the need to share the extraordinary care that this L&D team provided, and to remind myself… and you… why we became nurses… to touch, to heal, and to make a difference in the lives of others.

~Leanne Sells

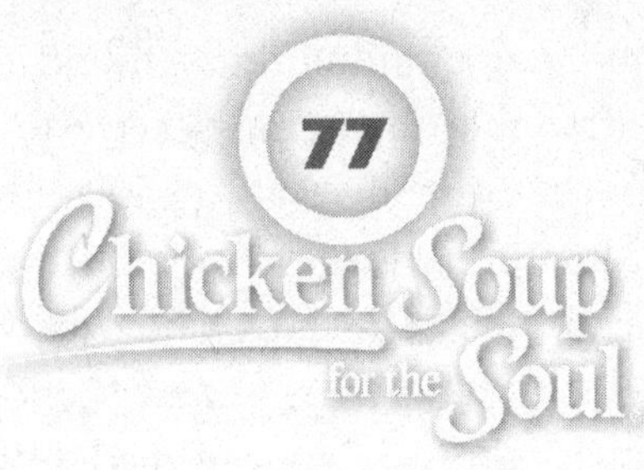

A Nurse's Sixth Sense

Walking with a friend in the dark is better than walking alone in the light.
~Helen Keller

They weren't even on call, those nurses who saved me. I was just coming in from my appointment with the orthopedic specialist, feeling excited and terrified, when I scurried to answer the phone on the last ring. At age thirty-three, after a lifelong struggle with an arthritic hip, I had just scheduled hip replacement surgery.

"Kathy, this is Mary Lu," said my nurse-friend whom I hadn't seen in months. "I've been thinking about you and wondering, have you decided what to do about that bad hip of yours?"

Our paths didn't cross often because she was a dynamic, highly successful nurse, wife, and mother of two. She was too busy for casual phone chats, and today was no exception. Yet, from out of the blue, this intuitive, compassionate nurse somehow knew I was getting ready to change my life.

Fast-forward twenty-two years. That hip I received in 1985 did in fact change my life. It gave me years of pain-free mobility before it wore out and was replaced by a second prosthesis.

On the day I was being discharged from the hospital, the nurses were changing my dressings and I gasped in pain. Just then the phone rang. It was Mary Lu. When she heard my tears, she spoke softly, directing me to think about the warm sunshine I'd soon be feeling.

Unfortunately, I contracted a severe staph infection. The pain in that prosthetic hip took me to the limit of my endurance. "Oh God," I prayed, "I need more strength. I need more help. I need more!"

That's when the card from Mary Lu arrived in the mail. In my weakened state I could barely read it. I smiled at her kind note. But as I placed it on the nightstand a tiny inscription on the back called out to me. *I have come that you may have life, and have it abundantly*.

And there it was. This nurse-friend had sent me a card that bore, on the very back and in the tiniest print, the answer to my agonizing prayer. I had prayed for more strength, and I knew down deep in my aching bones, that God was going to give it to me abundantly.

On a chilly November day, Mary Lu came by to see me. My nervous system was badly shaken because of the infection and I sometimes spent whole days just weeping. Mary Lu wrapped me in warm clothes and navigated my wheelchair out into the back yard, winter-cold and gray. We sat in silence. Then she pointed at a bird on the wire above the house. "Listen, Kathy. Can you hear what your little friend up there is saying? 'You're going to be well. You are going to be strong. God is here. You are utterly safe.'"

And I have felt utterly safe from that day forward. How did Mary Lu know to call, and to write, and to come, and to speak the perfect words when she did?

The intuitive compassion of other nurse-friends continued to astound me.

Karen was a powerhouse nurse at a labor and delivery hospital. One night, somehow sensing that my husband Ben couldn't stay awake with me one more hour, she arrived at the hospital, put her sleeping bag down on the floor, and huddled with me for the long night of bright lights, 2 a.m. blood draws, and my endless weeping. How on earth did she know I would need her so desperately that night?

A few weeks later, when I was home, Karen and our friend Patty came to visit. Ben played the piano as they sang the comforting carols that are the soundtrack of my life. I tried to sit up straight and be strong and grateful. The minute Ben left for work Karen's whole affect changed. "Okay, Kathy, you did great. You were strong. You gave Ben the comfort he needed in order to leave you and go to work. Now lie down and I'll give you a massage." Tears of gratitude and relief poured out from me. As she gently massaged my neck she soothed, "You are so tired of this pain. You are so weary from the struggle. It's okay. Just let it all out. It's okay to cry. I'm crying with you." How did she know the touch and words I needed?

Laura, the outstanding emergency room nurse, brought wonderfully nourishing meals and patiently helped me navigate my crutches through the mall at Christmastime. How did she know that my beauty-starved soul needed to be fed with music and lights?

Jean, my lifelong nurse-friend, lived in Anchorage and was monitoring my many hospitalizations with growing distress. Intuitively, she called me and immediately assessed that I was losing ground quickly. She questioned why no surgery date had been set for the dreaded placement of the new hip. Jean called my surgeon and discovered that he was unaware of my weakening state; I had been too ill to keep his office appraised. He immediately scheduled the surgery because in ten days he was leaving the country for several months. If Jean hadn't made that call, I know without a doubt I would never have endured until his return. Given my complicated medical history, he was the only doctor in the region who could perform this surgery. How did she know her call would save my life?

They weren't even on duty, these nurses. They were beloved friends. But they each possessed that unique sixth sense, the supernatural gift of great nurses. They sheltered me safely back to my life. And I have lived it abundantly ever since.

~Kathy McGovern

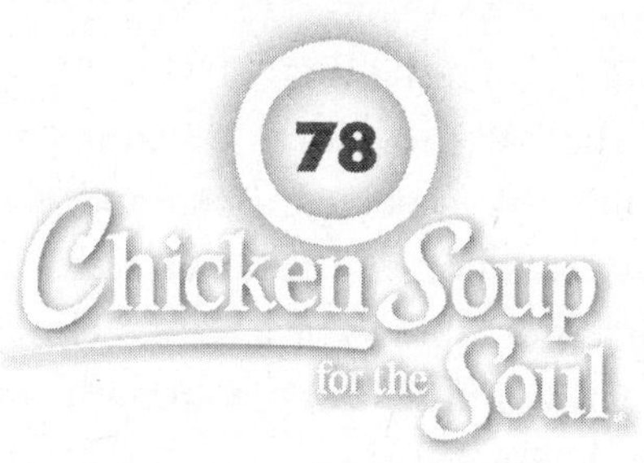

The Book Group

A mistake is to commit a misunderstanding.
~Bob Dylan

It was a surgery like any other, over and done with, and we were waiting for our patient to awake from his dreamland before transferring him into the recovery room. However, he seemed perfectly happy to sleep. So we waited, and waited, and waited some more.

As the minutes ticked by, the operating room staff began to engage in talk about current events such as the weather, who was on call for the weekend, and the latest Stephanie Plum book.

We all had our favorite characters. The nurse anesthetist liked Grandma, with her tight sausage head curls, continuous social visits to the funeral home, and the frankness that came with her age. The surgical technician preferred Stephanie herself, the bail-bonds woman and her trouble capturing her law-breaking surety, plus the hot men in her life. As for me, I liked Lula, an ex-prostitute. She was a greater-than-average woman with a large-size personality to boot. She wore tight, colorful, crazy outfits and had a love of food, especially the drive-through kind.

As we discussed the exploits in the newest book, the characters came alive. Time passed and the nurse anesthetist finally said we could transfer the patient. Although there was still no movement, we headed toward the recovery room, with the anesthetist pushing the gurney and me pulling from the foot.

Halfway down the hall the patient sat straight up like a mummy rising from his tomb. His eyes were open and glazed over, but still looking like nobody was home. Staring straight at me, he declared, "You gave up being a prostitute to be a nurse? How admirable. Thank you." He closed his eyes and lowered himself into the tomb from whence he came.

I was horrified; my mouth dropped open. If I'd had a heart condition I surely would have gone into V-fib. The anesthetist stood, speechless.

I often wonder what that patient remembers. Did he think it was only a drug-induced dream? Or a vision of a girl who gave up the red light district to carry the white lamp of Florence Nightingale, still caring for the needs of others, but in a very different way?

~Judy Mae Benson

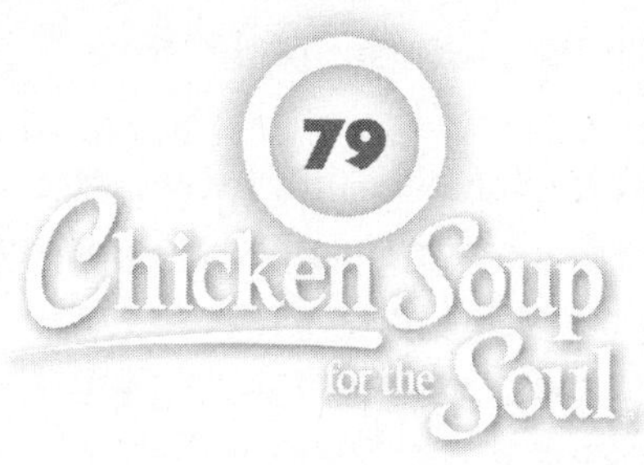

Person of the Year

God's dream is that you and I and all of us will realize that we are family, that we are made for togetherness, for goodness, and for compassion.
~Desmond Tutu

"Ebola Healthcare Workers Are Dying Faster Than Their Patients" read the *TIME* headline on October 3, 2014. *Forbes* stated the following week, "Ebola Has Killed More Than 200 Doctors, Nurses and Other Healthcare Workers Since June," citing that the two major countries affected were Sierra Leone and Liberia.

Sad. Frightening. But far away. In Africa. Far away, that was, until I received the phone call.

My son Paul had been working in a federal prison in California as a nurse practitioner when he was asked to become part of a Rapid Development Force (RDF) with the United States Public Health Service. USPHS is one of the seven active duty uniformed services; the other six are the Army, Air Force, Navy, Marines, Coast Guard, and NOAA (National Oceanic and Atmospheric Administration.) With USPHS he would join healthcare professionals sent to aid in situations such as natural diseases, world health crises, and to provide medical support for enormous crowds, like a presidential inauguration.

I was happy that Paul was part of this team, until the Ebola crisis hit.

The media reported that healthcare workers were being transported back to the States for treatment. Some lived; others didn't. We watched and prayed for them as we learned more details about this little-known plague. Fear swept throughout the nation and signs began to appear asking those entering from certain countries to be denied access.

President Obama, at the request of the United Nations, ordered the Surgeon General of the U.S. to activate seventy workers in the USPHS to travel to Liberia to set up and treat healthcare workers infected with the Ebola virus. Paul was among those contacted. Of course he would go. Any of the seventy could have declined, yet none did. Paul's group would be the first team sent.

After a weeklong stateside training by the Center for Disease Control in Aniston, Alabama, they would fly to Liberia on October 26th to begin their two-month mission.

It's one thing to see disaster on the news, but another to realize that your son is going to put himself directly in harm's way. "Be anxious for nothing," I kept saying to myself, remembering Philippians 4:6, "but in everything by prayer and supplication with thanksgiving let your requests be made known to God." I tried.

On my way to prayer on Saturday morning, after a sleepless night, while waiting for the traffic signal to change. I sensed in my spirit that small voice. "Haven't you been praying for these people?" I had. "Well, I'm trying to send them help." I began to feel some peace.

Through the days that followed, I thought of Paul. He would continue his work at the prison until Friday, then have two days to prepare. He was told to update his will and insurance benefits, make funeral arrangements, purchase scrubs, mosquito netting… the list continued. As a single dad with grown sons, he lived alone in California. There would be no one there to say goodbye. My heart ached. I just couldn't let that happen. Of course I flew to California.

Paul met me at the airport on Thursday evening and for the next two days we worked feverishly. By Sunday morning he was packed and ready. I snapped pictures of him as he hauled his two large bags toward his boarding gate. He didn't look back.

The seventy volunteers that convened in Alabama included not only doctors and nurses, but lab technicians, photographers, scientists, writers, psychologists, chaplains, and engineers. For a week they learned safety procedures and practiced donning and doffing Hazmat suits for protection. The more the team learned, the more confident they felt.

But the somber headlines continued. A traveler from Liberia tested positive in Texas and died. The more news reports we heard, the more anxious our country became.

That Saturday we said our goodbyes over the phone. Paul was ready.

The team arrived in Liberia to find field hospitals set up by the military. Supplies began arriving and they stocked shelves. While recovering from jet lag and adjusting to the extreme heat and humidity, they met with Doctors Without Borders and were greeted by the Liberian President and the Minister of Health. President Obama called and spoke with the team and eventually the Secretary General of the UN toured the facility.

A week after being there, their first patient, a healthcare worker named Alvin, arrived. Paul led him from the ambulance to the makeshift hospital, started his IV, drew labs, and administrated medication.

Although these volunteers were more than 5,000 miles from home, the Internet, texting, and even FaceTime allowed us to feel like we were part of the action. The more we learned, the more our anxiety lessened.

We all celebrated when Alvin was released. When Paul's team removed the protective gear from their faces, Alvin saw, for the first time, the caregivers who he had jokingly referred to as Spacemen. A ceremony was held and Alvin received a certificate declaring him to be Ebola free. Outside the tent a hand-painted makeshift board read, "Today I am Healed. Tomorrow I Return to Heal Another." Each patient who survived would leave his or her handprint on the board. When Alvin became the third his family cheered. Soon he would return to his medical practice, immune to the virus, to treat his own Ebola patients.

Throughout the next several weeks the teams rotated shifts. Nurses and doctors worked sixteen hours, two hours in full protective garb with temperatures inside the uniform soaring to 115 degrees. Another three hours were spent rehydrating and sleeping.

More handprints were added to the board, each one representing another healthcare provider saved. Those who didn't survive were photographed for their families, placed in body bags, and sent for burial.

A week before Paul's team returned home, the second group of USPHS volunteers arrived to be trained. Already word had begun to spread to caregivers in neighboring African countries that help was nearby. With the news that they would have a place to go if they became infected, large numbers of healthcare workers once again returned to Liberia to fight this dreadful disease.

Ebola is no longer the lead story on the evening news. Ebola rates have dropped dramatically in Liberia, though it is far from cured.

The real heroes in this story are those men and women who daily train and serve both here and abroad, putting their lives at risk to serve others. No wonder *TIME* named these Ebola fighters their Person of the Year for 2014.

~Phyllis Bird Nordstrom

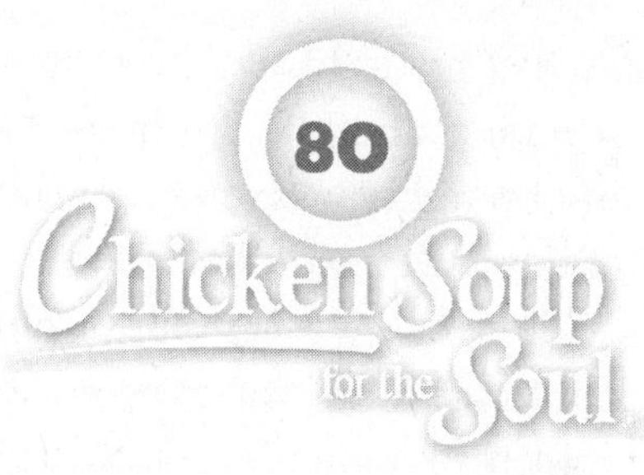

Touching Hearts

There is something in the nature of things which the mind of man, which reason, which human power cannot effect, and certainly that which produces this must be better than man.
~Cicero

I was working as a nurse in a surgery department for a small community hospital when I attended a Sunday evening service where missionaries presented stories of their work in foreign countries. I knew then I needed to use my nursing skills in some type of missionary work. I found a wonderful organization through my church, and signed on for a trip.

I'd never been away from my wife for any length of time, had never flown in a large airplane, and was nervous about traveling to another country. My anxiety heightened when we arrived in Honduras. We rode four-and-a-half hours on an old school bus and stopped at a police checkpoint. Our translator cautioned us not to take pictures and to stay on the bus. We finally continued our journey and arrived at a motel where a man stood guard with an automatic rifle. Our leader immediately began searching for a safer place to stay. My heart thumped. I had never been exposed to anything like this before, but I knew I had a calling to work in a medical clinic in this dangerous territory.

But first we had to build one. The first two days, we medical volunteers assisted the volunteer construction team in building a clinic.

The local Hondurans had made blocks from clay and laid them in the sun to dry. Constructing a building from the blocks and working in the intense heat and humidity was tough, physically and mentally.

After a couple of days, we medical volunteers traveled to other communities to provide care. Two Honduran physicians accompanied us. I was shocked to see hundreds of people lined up in hope of accessing care for problems ranging from malnutrition to infections. They looked at us as if we were superstars, though I'm sure they were snickering at my Southern-drawl Spanish. Through the heat and labor, it was great to be needed and appreciated.

One community, once ravaged by a hurricane, had a sign at the main entrance with flags from various countries that had funded its rebuilding. Now people in tiny clay-block homes had access to outhouses and a water tower. Kids were running around playing games.

We set up a makeshift clinic in a one-room church building there. The windows were actually holes covered by large pieces of removable plywood. Tables near the front of the church held medications. In one corner, two curtains were hung to make two exam rooms. Crowds started pouring into the church. The temperature was scorching that day and there was no breeze despite the open windows.

I assisted one of the physicians in the hot exam room. A young boy, probably six or seven years old, was escorted by his mother, who began talking to the Honduran doctor in Spanish. The doctor examined the boy and listened to his chest with a stethoscope. He suddenly stopped and said to me in English, "This boy has a heart murmur so large you can feel it by placing a hand on his chest." As I did so, I was astounded to feel the swishing of the blood through the hole in this little boy's heart.

The physician said softly, "There are no facilities here for this child to have surgery or any medical intervention." He frowned. "All we can do is pray."

Instinctively, I placed my hand on the boy's chest again, this time to pray to God for his healing. The physician joined in Spanish as fervently as I prayed in English. Then I felt something I had never felt before and I have never felt again. An electrical shock initiated at the top of my head and jolted through my arm and then left my hand. I was overwhelmed with emotion and the strong feeling of God's presence.

After soft words of explanation and limited medical directives, the boy and his mother left our clinic. We completed our day and I couldn't wait to tell the other volunteers about my life-changing event. As we rode our bus back to the hotel, I eagerly recounted my experience. One group member said, "Wait until you hear what we experienced at the exact same time!"

The hot humid air had been stifling in the church, he said. The plywood windows were open but there was no air movement. As more people gathered in the church, it got even hotter. "We heard you praying behind the curtain. Just then a breeze began to blow in the church, but it wasn't coming from the windows or the open doors. We looked toward your exam room and saw the sheet blowing outward there! We, too, all felt the presence of God."

The Great Physician touched many hearts that week, perhaps mine most of all.

~Jeff Radford

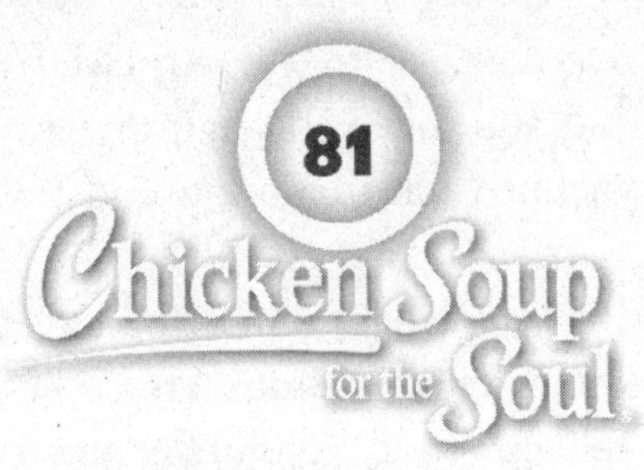

Jane Doe

Act as if what you do makes a difference. It does.
~William James

Jane Doe was a sixty-year-old woman found unconscious outside a gas station and brought by EMS to our level one trauma center in Philadelphia. Her total down time was well over thirty minutes before she finally arrived at the ICU, where I was assigned as her primary nurse. She had already been intubated, was on three vasopressors, and about to begin emergent dialysis treatment. They had aborted the hypothermic protocol due to her instability and poor prognosis.

The next morning I returned to learn Jane had lost brainstem reflexes overnight, and doctors were beginning the brain death protocol. At that moment I realized I was all Jane had at the end of her life. No one knew who she was or where she was from. As she lay in the hospital bed dying, I began to wonder, was Jane a mother, a sibling, a spouse, or a grandmother to someone who was out searching and praying for her safe return home? Would they be reunited before she passed away?

I made it my goal to reunite Jane with her loved ones. She didn't have much time on earth, so I had to keep her alive until her family could be located. I sorted through her belongings to see if I could piece together the puzzle of who Jane actually was. An unopened

Pepsi bottle and pack of cigarettes with a receipt from the gas station was all I found in her possession. I went back out to the nurse's station and called the phone number on the receipt, thinking maybe she frequented there and they might know her name. The number was out of order.

It was a Saturday morning and I knew there was probably only one social worker on call, but Jane deserved this effort so I had to try. When the social worker returned my call, he told me his colleague handled the unknown identity patients and would be back in on Monday. He said he was already busy handling all of the discharges for the day.

I pleaded with him. "You have to help me solve this mystery. This woman most likely won't be alive on Monday." I began to cry. "It is both of our professional responsibilities to help patients and their loved ones in their greatest time of need and vulnerability. And this is one of those times. The discharges can wait."

"I will help you," he offered. "I'll contact the Philadelphia Police Department and arrange for them to come and fingerprint her."

By noon, a police officer walked onto the unit looking for me. After explaining Jane's condition, he promised he would try his best. He even said he would go out into the community and knock on doors to see if anyone could help in our investigation. His shift was over at 3:00 p.m., and if he did not have any luck he would pass it on to the next officer on duty.

As he left, Jane's blood pressure began to drop and there was nothing else medically we could do to help her. Her time was running out.

It was only an hour later when the officer returned with her identity. He had knocked on a door down the street from the gas station. Someone there was able to identify Jane based on his description. It turned out Jane was indeed important to many. She was a single mother of four, an older sister, and a grandmother to six beautiful children.

The doctors contacted the family, who quickly came to be by

her side. They surrounded her bed and prayed, and she passed away minutes later.

Jane must have been waiting for them to find her before she put her feet on heaven's stairway.

~Amanda Conley

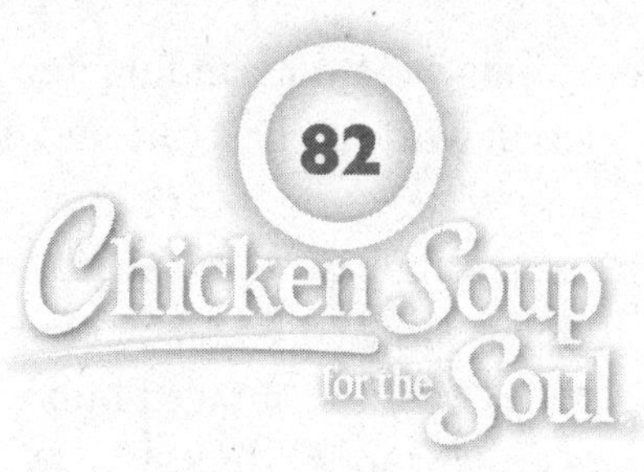

Dad's "Girls"

Work is love made visible.
~Kahlil Gibran

I had a pressing dilemma. My widowed father was diagnosed with late-stage lung cancer, and it was left to me to care for him. My siblings had careers; my career was as a childcare provider in my home.

I had eight children, from newborn to five years, in my care from about 6:30 a.m. until 6:30 p.m. every weekday. I had to believe there was a way for me to care for them and care for Dad too.

Three of my childcare parents called my father "Grandad," as I had provided care for them when they were little children. They were adamant that I take my dad into my home and care for him. They wanted their children to be able to love him, and to experience the passing of an older person before it got "too close to home."

Three of my childcare moms were nurses. By Divine coincidence, two were geriatric nurses, the third one an oncology nurse. Just what I needed.

While my dad was still in the hospital, I had a conference with my childcare parents. Their overwhelming support for Dad and me was amazing. I moved him into our home and some of his greatest pleasure during his last days was watching and interacting with the little children who adored him. Seeing their youth, innocence, and vibrancy helped him deal with his pain.

While all of the parents were outstanding during this time, "my" nurses were truly angels in white in their care and nurturing of Dad… and my family and me.

When I couldn't make him use his oxygen, one of them came after work and knelt down so he could see her face. She sweet talked him into trying the oxygen and encouraged him with gentleness. He grew to love her. "She understands why I have to use this stuff more than the rest of you put together!" She came into my home every evening, exhausted from her twelve-hour shifts. Yet she greeted her children, then visited with my dad, checking his vitals, going over the handwritten medical charts I kept for him, and telling him funny stories as she hovered over him.

Another parent, the oncology nurse, the one with the emotionally draining career, reinforced with me how to become comfortable with the valve drain procedure. We had a hospice nurse for Dad, which I appreciated so very much, but this nurse helped me a couple of times so he didn't have to leave the house in the middle of a cold Colorado winter. She kept me abreast of his symptoms and the progression of his disease. It was so edifying to be able to understand the changes happening to him and the emotions she knew he was dealing with. It was such a comfort to know she would be there every day.

The third nurse, who was the most personally caring person I'd ever met, spent time nurturing me and my family and our holistic health. She brought dinner several times and even ordered pizza when she was too exhausted to prepare a meal for us. She cautioned me, my husband, and our fifteen-year-old son to take care of ourselves, to deal with the situation as it progressed, to talk openly about what was happening, to share with her and with one another the trauma we were all going through.

My daycare children, my other childcare parents, and my entire family benefitted greatly from the ministry of these three nurses. My brothers and sister living far away were comforted knowing I had daily professional help with Dad. The nurses watched for any indication of stress the little children might be experiencing. They talked with my son, asking him if he had questions or concerns, challenging him to be open and honest about his feelings. They answered our questions and explained Dad's progression towards death. They matter-of-factly shared stories with Dad about their dealings with terminal patients.

For two months, each one of them gave totally of themselves, after an exhausting workday, knowing they had small children to care for, meals to prepare, laundry to do, a house to clean, and a husband to share with after they left my home. Not one of them ever complained. Not one of them ever rushed through picking up her children. Not one of them ever expressed impatience.

They gave me a chance to breathe, sometimes for the first time that day. Even in his pain, Dad looked forward to their arrival each day. For him it was a chance to see "his girls" as he called them, freely sharing how he felt emotionally as well as physically.

One nurse picked her child up late one evening because she'd had a death on her unit. She cried softly in my arms about losing one of her patients.

We lost Dad ten minutes after she left.

I would not have been able to care for him and the children without the love and ministry of "Dad's girls," his angels in white. To quote Dad, "There are special places in heaven for 'girls' like mine."

~Bette Haywood Matero

Keepsake

Keep all special thoughts and memories for lifetimes to come. Share these keepsakes with others to inspire hope and build from the past, which can bridge to the future.
~Mattie Stepanek

Mom had beautiful hair. From an early age, she loved trying out different styles and trends. Looking at pictures of her from childhood to middle age was like thumbing through a hair-styling magazine in a beauty salon.

When she was diagnosed with brain cancer at the age of forty-eight, our family was devastated. Mom was especially dismayed when the neurosurgeon told her they would have to shave her head in the operating room.

My mother was a simple woman, born and raised in the foothills of Ohio in the 1940s. Times were tough and she enjoyed few luxuries growing up. But the one thing she treasured and spent considerable time and effort on was her hair.

As a small child, she sported a short pixie cut with razor-straight bangs. Then came barrettes and hairbands in grade school. As a teenager, she graduated to long brunette locks with a side part and gorgeous waves. She was rocking the Cindy Crawford look before Cindy was even born.

My mother never finished high school. At seventeen, she met my father, who was a submarine sailor in the United States Navy. After a whirlwind courtship they eloped, and over the next thirty-one years, my father took my mother all over the world and did his best to spoil her.

One of her favorite ways to pamper herself was going to a hair salon, something her family couldn't afford when she was young. Over the years, there were pin curls and perms, bouffants and bobs, and an unfortunate wedge in the 1980s that Mom couldn't grow out fast enough. The one thing she didn't do to her hair was change the color. Her dark mahogany brown was a prettier shade than anything from a bottle, with auburn highlights in the summer from days spent on the beach and gardening in the sun. She gave in a bit however in her forties — "just a wash" — to cover those dreaded grays.

The night before her surgery, I spent extra time with Mom, brushing her thick luxurious hair while she shed more than a few tears.

After her operation, she woke up in the intensive care unit with a blue surgical bonnet covering her head. Once she got her bearings, the first thing she did was yank off the bonnet and ask for a mirror. She stared at her reflection for a long time, gingerly running a hand over her bare head, careful not to touch the railroad track of staples and sutures on the right side. Then she dropped the mirror on the bed and asked us to put the cap back on.

"It'll grow back," I reassured her.

In her drug-induced stupor, she only nodded and said, "Okay."

A nurse came into the room and handed my father a clear plastic bag. "The scrub nurse in the OR saved this for you."

It was Mother's hair.

I don't know what prompted the nurse to do that — no one asked her to — but I'm so incredibly glad she did. Contrary to our hopes, the subsequent chemo and radiation treatments left Mom with permanent hair loss; only a few wispy strands grew back. My father spared no expense in finding her two of the finest wigs money could buy. But it wasn't the same.

Mother lost her battle to cancer a year later, but I still have a piece of her with me. I've kept it for more than twenty years now, wrapped in tissue paper and tucked away in my bureau drawer. Once in while I take it out, and the scent of Mom comes back to me all over again, reminding me of my wonderful childhood and mother.

It's not your typical keepsake, but it means more to me than the trinkets or jewelry or any material possession Mom handed down to me. I am so thankful to that scrub nurse who thought to sweep this treasure from the OR floor.

~Cheryll Snow

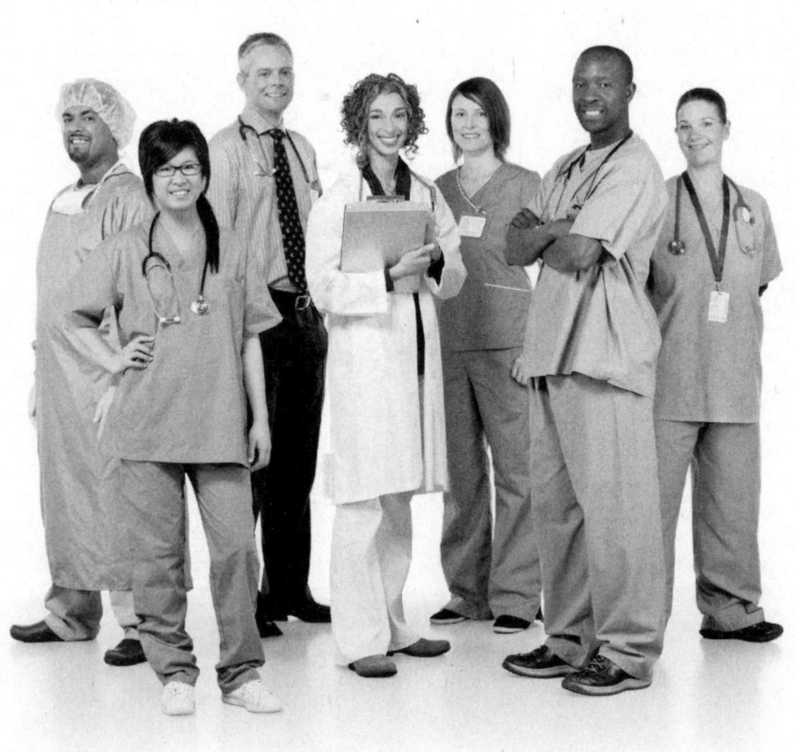

Inspiration for Nurses

Heart of a Nurse

It is an absolute human certainty that no one can know his own beauty or perceive a sense of his own worth until it has been reflected back to him in the mirror of another loving, caring human being.

~John Joseph Powell

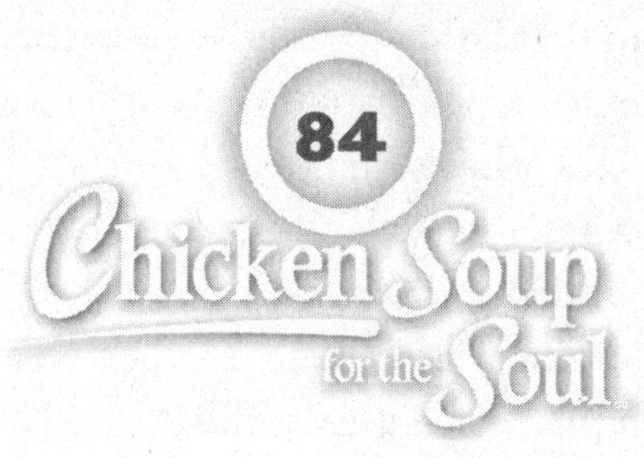

Tender Hands

There never was any heart truly great and generous, that was not also tender and compassionate.
~Robert Frost

My mama's bright, flowered scrubs were spattered with dried blood as she came through the door of her little house. My older sister Andrea followed Mama in, wearing her own bright scrubs, sunshine yellow covered with scampering turtles. I was at my parents' to check in on Daddy, recently home from the hospital himself. As they came toward the kitchen, Andrea grinned at me and asked in her big Southern accent, "Is there coffee?"

I laughed. In this house of healthcare professionals, with long shifts the norm, coffee flowed like air. "You know there is."

I poured them both a cup as they dropped their big work bags, the ones they packed in the early dark hours, putting in whatever they needed for the long shifts they worked as nurses in eastern North Carolina.

Andrea had become a nurse in her twenties, while taking care of her own kids. Mama, on the other hand, got her nursing degree much later, after raising the tribe of us, when she had "finally gotten us grown enough to dress ourselves and pour our own cereal." She went to the local community college and had been proudly pinned at forty-nine, beginning the career she had dreamed of her whole life.

Now, they left in the dark and they came home in the dark. They still wore their stethoscopes hanging around their necks as they dropped into the ladder-back chairs at Mama's table, laughing and talking. I brought a mug of coffee for each of them and pulled out my own chair to join them. Pretty much my whole family worked in health care… my mother, sister, and brother were nurses, another sister worked in the pharmaceutical industry, and my dad had retired from a career at an alcoholic rehab center. I had studied English in college, so I listened in awe to the stories of life and death situations my family encountered every day.

Once, a few years before, when I had first started college, I had sat with them as I did now, listening as they had talked about a patient in cardiac arrest, one they had worked to "bring back." I had cried, saying, "Y'all do real work! You save lives! What am I doing studying English? You're so noble!" Then I had added, "Maybe I should become a nurse."

They had both burst into laughter, Mama saying, "Honey, you can't change the cat box without getting sick." Andrea giggled as Mama told me, "You'll find what you're supposed to do. Nursing is not for everyone."

Now, several years later, as they shook off the long day at the nursing home, I thought about it again. Whatever I ended up doing, I wanted to love it as much they did. I wanted to have as much passion and get as much satisfaction as they did. And that passion was clear no matter what kind of nursing they did.

They had both done hospital nursing—cardiology, oncology, infectious diseases, emergency services. They also did home health care. Mama was even one of the first nurses in our county to care for AIDS patients in the eighties. They had worked as travel nurses a few times, flying to various places—San Francisco was Mama's favorite—to work in dire situations where nurses were needed.

But the work they both loved best, the work they had devoted the bulk of their careers to, was caring for long-term care patients, those closest to the end of their lives, the beautiful old men and women spending their final days, months, sometimes years in skilled nursing facilities. "My little old people," Mama said, making me laugh because many of them were younger than she was.

She and Andrea both regularly packed their bags with those stethoscopes, favorite bandage scissors, the personal equipment their jobs required, but also with treats for the elders in their care—Andes candies for the little man with a sweet tooth, a garden tomato for the bedridden woman whose eyes still lit up when she talked of gardening, a fleece cap with a pretty flower for the woman whose thinning hair left her embarrassed and cold, a birthday cake and card to be signed for the man whose family seldom visited. They always had something planned: Mama's silly paper crown of red hearts for Valentine's Day, tiny Andrea standing only 4'10" dressing up as an elf around Christmas, the two of them packing books for the readers, or clothes for patients who came in with little. Care for them meant tending to their spirits as well as their aging fragile bodies. But those fragile bodies made it difficult for me to understand how these women I loved did what they did every day.

As many days as they came home happy, they also came home somber, sadness wreathing their eyes as they returned quiet from long shifts, made even longer by the death of a patient to whom they gave their days—and their hearts.

Now, sipping her coffee, Mama's smile faded as she asked Andrea if she had looked in on one particular patient. My sister nodded, her own bright eyes darkening. They both always honored the confidentiality of their patients; even so, I understood immediately they were anticipating a death.

Andrea circled the big mug with her small hands, and murmured, "Won't be long."

"The family all know?" Mama asked.

Andrea nodded, and silence settled between them. I sputtered, "How—how do you do it?"

They looked up at me surprised. "Do what?" Mama asked.

I shook my head, tearful. "How can you stand it? I mean, your patients always die!" I looked back and forth between them. "How does it not break your heart?"

Andrea smiled softly, and said. "Everyone dies, baby girl."

I still couldn't grasp it, how they kept so positive, tucking mints and cards into their bags when every day, any day, someone they'd taken care of for months, even years, could die.

"But—but, I don't understand..." Crying now, I couldn't even ask the question.

Mama slid her chair closer, placing her hand over mine. "It is hard, harder sometimes than others."

I looked up into her blue eyes. "Why would you put yourself through that?"

She stroked my hair, and said, "You know, if you think about it, there's always so much celebration, so many tender hands, when we come into this world."

My sister looked across the table at me with kind eyes.

Mama patted my hand, and said, "We do this work, even when it breaks our hearts, because we think..." She wiped a tear from my cheek and smiled. "We think there should be tender hands when we leave this world, too."

I nodded, but I didn't say anything. Mama had said everything there was to say.

~Mary Carroll-Hackett

Privileged Presence

Therefore, comfort each other and edify one another, just as you are doing.
~1 Thessalonians 5:11

I was a member of the Rapid Response Team. I had just finished rounds and returned to my home unit. I was cruising through the Surgery Intensive Care Unit to check if anyone needed help when I'd noticed the crash cart outside Room 20 and a flurry of activity inside. "Prime the Levophed line and get Bicarb STAT!" I rushed to get the Bicarb when I was nearly run down by a coworker.

"Aren't you the family-centered care person? This young man's mom is on the phone, wailing. Please help."

I asked someone else to get the Bicarb, and I approached the phone feeling very nervous. I had never met this woman and knew little about her son, except that he was twenty years old and was expected to die soon.

I took a deep breath and looked upward, wishing for some Divine intervention. What could I possibly say? I picked up the phone. "Hi, my name is Mary. I am one of the nurses here. I'm answering for Kim because she is with Michael."

The woman on the other end cried, "The doctor called and said my son is dying right now! I am four hours away. Is this true?"

"I am sorry, yes, he is in big trouble. We are doing our best to keep him alive. I don't know you and this is awful information to be giving you on the phone. I am so sorry."

"What am I going to do? This can't happen! I don't want him to die without me."

My heart was racing. Even as a well-seasoned nurse, experienced with many patient death situations, I was numb and at a loss for words. I said, "I am so sorry. We're doing everything we can. I'll stay on the phone with you." Then the Divine intervention I had been praying for came. I remembered that our unit clerks had cordless phones at their desks. I heard myself say, "I am going to take the phone to your son. I'll put it to his ear and you can talk to him. I will talk with you every few minutes and let you know what we are doing."

"Okay," she said.

On my way to the room, I explained that we were giving drugs for his blood pressure and continuing to try everything.

"Can he hear me?" she asked.

"Yes, I believe he can hear everything, even though he can't respond to you." I encouraged her to say all she had in her heart and felt was important. "Talk about any unfinished issues or just tell him you love him."

As the next forty minutes passed, I stayed next to the bed with the phone pressed to her son's ear. Michael was in full-blown arrest and the code continued furiously around me. Every few minutes I spoke with Mom and updated her on Michael's heart rate, chest compressions, blood pressure, and drugs given. During this time, his dad called and I put another phone on the other ear, but this only lasted for a few minutes. The dad lived about forty-five minutes away and decided to try and make it to the hospital.

As things became increasingly dismal and it was time to call the code, I told the mother that Michael's heart rate was now very slow, not really beating right at all, and that this was the end. I put the phone back to his ear as she spoke her final words to her son.

One minute later Michael was asystolic and the code was called. I had been crying for a while already. Brokenhearted, I told her Michael was gone.

Our attending MD took the phone, offered her condolences and answered questions. Kim, Michael's nurse, also talked with her. I spoke with her one last time.

She sobbed, "Thank you for helping me be with him. You'll never know what it meant to me…." Her voice broke.

Still feeling helpless and inadequate, I had a tearful decompression with my coworkers. They helped me realize the difference I had made, and understood my bittersweet feelings of privileged presence.

We nurses are given a great gift to provide help and comfort to people in their darkest hours. Privileged indeed.

~Mary Gagnon

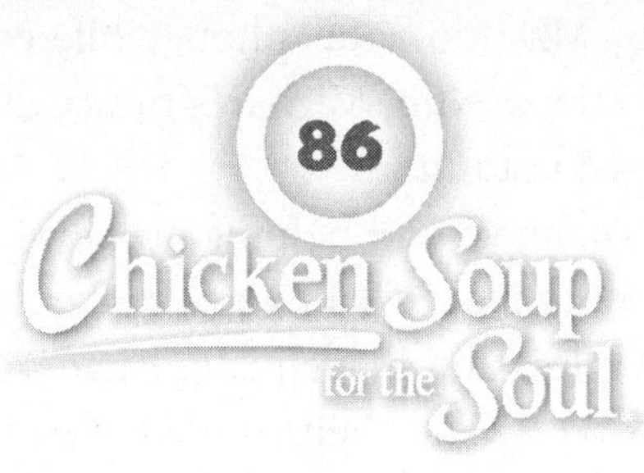

Body, Mind and Spirit

One word frees us of all the weight and pain of life: that word is love.
~Sophocles

I found her husband in a chair with his upper body draped over the bed, his head on the mattress next to hers. I unintentionally startled him when I walked into the room and apologized.

"I'm Doug, Kay's nurse tonight," I said softly. "I'm going to do her assessment and give the scheduled medications. We're trying to stabilize her heart rate and blood pressure."

Kay was just twenty-six, with multiple myeloma, now on a ventilator and heavily sedated to manage her pain and restlessness.

As I performed my routine duties, I noticed Mike was obviously fatigued and the redness around his eyes proved he'd been crying. He had that perplexed look on his face, the one that's apparent on those who recognize the outcome for their loved ones isn't going to be what they hoped.

They had been married for less than two years and had no children. I didn't know if that was good or bad. A part of me wished that a child had been born to serve as a living reminder of their love. Another part of me thought that in the absence of a child, it might be easier for him to start over when the time was right. I felt the loneliness and sheer devastation he was feeling and wished there was something I could do to make a difference. But how could I?

Body, mind and spirit, I reminded myself. These were the interdependent domains toward which I had always directed my work. So, when I no longer could affect healing of the body, I focused more sharply on the mind and spirit.

Also, I saw family as an extension of the patient, a reflection of the patient's identity, his or her feelings, emotions, values and beliefs. Family, however defined, became the voice of the patient and served as a barometer of acceptance.

The energy in the room changed as Kay's fate became increasingly clearer. Mike had recently appeared more confused, distressed and detached. Then it occurred to me. They likely hadn't slept apart since they were married. So, after confirming this, I asked, "Mike, would you be comfortable sleeping with her now, keeping her safe, warm and connected to you?"

He looked stunned.

"I'll handle the logistics, manage the equipment and fend off the naysayers."

"Yes. Please," he said.

Within an hour of togetherness in their bed, there was yet another change in the energy in the room. This time there was peace and love. Kay's restlessness significantly diminished and that night she required fifty percent less sedation. She had fewer episodes of hypertension. Mike rested too, admitting a profound connectedness to her, emotionally and spiritually. The end no longer felt as cold, foreign or unwelcomed.

With this intentional caring of body, mind and spirit, the healing had begun.

~Doug Dascenzo

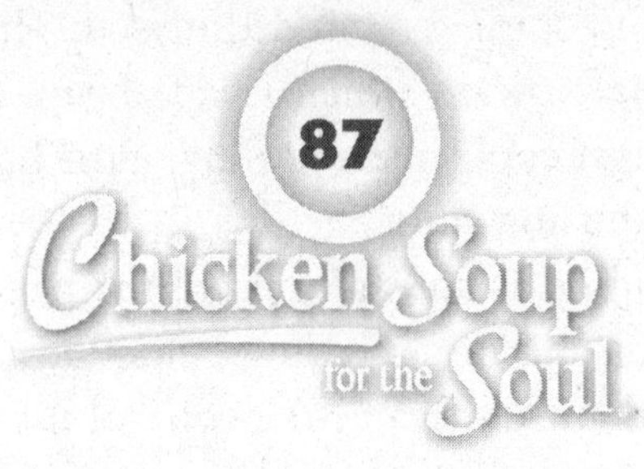

Nurse Sheila

No love, no friendship can cross the path of our destiny without leaving some mark on it forever.
~François Mauriac

My childhood friend Sheila attracted friendships easily with her warm, sincere and loving nature. And so too, she attracted me. We became pals when her family moved into the Veteran's Housing Development where I lived as a young girl in the early 1960s. During that time, many of our country's veterans took advantage of their well-earned G.I. benefits and stayed in the development just long enough to save money to buy a home. Others passed through as they waited for their next appointed military station. Some families like mine stayed. My father, having served our country during World War II, was happy to settle into the Veteran's Housing Project, where we put down roots and forged friendships. Sheila was mine.

We played together endlessly in the old neighborhood. Sheila was easy to be with and fun to be around. We shared the same interests and were in the same elementary school classrooms and Girl Scouts. Our lives meshed as we shared our secrets, dreams and aspirations.

But in time, to our great sadness, Sheila's family moved on, too. We said our goodbyes and promised to stay friends, but as so often happens in life, after a while we didn't keep in touch.

At age thirty-nine, out of the blue, I was diagnosed with Stage 2 breast cancer. This was a complete shock to me; I had no family history of cancer. I was a runner, a non-smoker and consumed little red meat. I drank a glass of wine only occasionally and overall took very good care of myself. “How could I have cancer?” I asked. I felt my body had betrayed me with this aggressive disease.

After the diagnosis, life as I knew it ended. The next few weeks were a whirlwind of endless tests, scans and blood work. I headed for surgery for a “wide excision lumpectomy” of my left breast. After an extended time in recovery, I was brought to my room.

Much later, when I opened my eyes, it took a minute to remember where I was. The room was dark except for a dim light illuminating the equipment hanging from the metal pole. I was surprised I’d slept at all. Nausea from the anesthesia was so wretched and violent, I wondered if I might not survive. I reached for the receptacle placed at my side and was comforted for a moment when my fingers found the cold stainless bowl.

“Can I do anything for you?” That’s all she said, so softly that I wondered at first if she had spoken at all. I turned and looked at the nurse who had been sitting so quietly in the dark. The soft glow of the light highlighted her blond hair and pleasant smile. I wondered how long she had been there.

She stood and took my hand in hers; her sweet smile was just as I remembered. “Hi Jackie, it’s me, Sheila.”

There were no words at first, just a knowing and fullness of what had once been. The years evaporated. Sheila stayed with me throughout the evening. She held my hair back when I got sick, then cleaned me up when I was done. We began sharing stories. Memories flooded back. The old familiar comfort felt reassuring. I cried as I mourned my breast and my health, while Sheila was empathetic, understanding, and strong.

Routinely she checked my vitals and my wound and managed my pain. Most of all, she listened as I sorted through and vented my fears for the future. We talked into the night. Sheila imparted her medical knowledge and cited positive examples of the many women she knew who had beaten breast cancer. She encouraged me to be strong and to fight. She praised the oncology department at the hospital. Eventually I fell asleep.

When I woke Sheila was gone, but remnants of the calmness she brought remained. I lay in the dimly lit room with only my thoughts. Our lives had once again meshed through our shared memories. Thanks to Sheila and her life-long warmth, sincerity and love, when dawn broke I greeted the new day and my future with an abundance of newfound hope… and friendship.

~Jacqueline Hickey

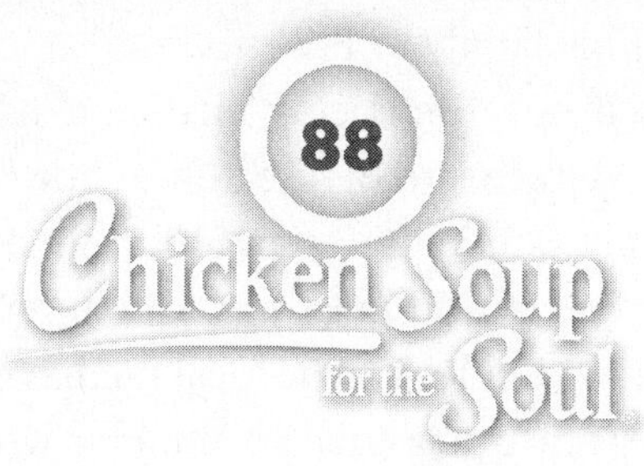

Surely You Know My Grandfather

Memories of our lives, of our works and our deeds will continue in others.
~Rosa Parks

My grandfather had been dead for twenty years by the time I needed to use his hospital. Most of the doctors he worked with had long since retired or passed away. I'm not even sure if his photograph still hung in any of the main hallways. But none of that stopped my mother from informing everybody about our family's legacy and general importance. After all, she was used to special treatment. My own birth had been overseen by the Chief of Staff in a private suite, and every rule had been broken to give her what she demanded. Apparently unaware that our celebrity status had expired, my mother greeted all of my nurses with, "This is Dr. Young's granddaughter."

Grandfather was an incredible man. Born and raised in rural Louisiana, he finished high school early, and went on to play football for Texas A&M. As a twenty-year-old college graduate, he was anxious to attend medical school, but was too young to apply. So, he did what any man would do in that situation—he played professional football for the Washington Redskins. He eventually became an OB/GYN, and after a stint in a small town to help a new hospital get its footing, he moved his family to Phoenix.

He kept himself busy practicing medicine, as well as serving as Chief of Staff and on the board of directors at one of the Valley's major hospitals, which my family still privately calls our own. His spare time was spent at Freemason meetings, where he held a respectable ranking. He was news fodder for the local media, which featured him frequently in a range of articles that covered his work for the hospital, as well as an entire piece dedicated to his large feet.

But life is more than a résumé, and my grandfather did not succeed at everything. He suffered from severe depression during a time when treatment involved shock therapy and numbing amounts of alcohol. His retirement was spent slumped in a recliner, remote in hand, and a never-ending game of football on the television five feet in front of him.

My family rarely mentioned him after his death. I didn't think of him often, until my mother began accosting nurses with his name.

The nurses would always smile brightly, nodding and writing on the whiteboard in front of my bed in big bubble letters with smiley faces. The really good ones would exclaim and press their hands to their hearts. My mother was decades out of date, but she maintained her resolve to find someone, anyone, who recognized his name.

On the day I was discharged, I had a new nurse. She was old, so old that I can only hope she was working due to love instead of need. I had to prove my ability to walk the hallway before I could earn my discharge papers, and she was there to serve as my witness. We set out for a record-setting walk, as I insisted on hobbling a step ahead of the elderly nurse so she wouldn't have to bear any of my weight.

My mother was waiting for us in my room, arriving just in time for one last bombardment. I shook my head, waiting for the professional eye roll the other nurses had mastered. But this nurse pushed back her hunched shoulders, folded her arms, and said, "Well, what do you know. I worked with Dr. Young." I thought Mom might explode with excitement.

The nurse sat next to me on my bed, poured herself a cup of water, and shared every memory she had of my grandfather. These weren't like the stories in the newspaper clippings I kept in my closet, or the staged moments that happened in the family photo album. She told me the stories we wanted to hear, the little details that explained why I don't like watermelon and use certain words. They were the stories I wish he could have told me himself.

"And one day, he had been sleeping in the bunks, when he burst out the door yelling for help. I was the only one there, so I rushed over, thinking there was some terrible emergency, and he told me I had to help him find his ring. He wore this very large, fancy ring...."

"It was a Freemason ring," my mother interrupted, her smile about to expand off her face.

"Yes, it was beautiful, and he had somehow lost it. We tore that room apart looking for it. He was such a large man and always walked proudly, so he looked very funny crawling around that dirty floor on all fours. I ended up finding the ring on the table next to his bunk. Imagine that! He was so relieved, and he couldn't stop thanking me."

I think she mistook my face's reaction to her story. Patting my hand, she stood, saying, "Well, I'd say you are fine to go home. You didn't need my help at all."

I still regret the lump in my throat that prevented me from speaking as she walked away. I wanted to tell her what her memories meant to me. I wanted to tell her that I had been walking by myself since yesterday anyway. I really wanted to tell her that I thought my grandfather was out there somewhere, thanking her still, for remembering him. I know Mother was.

~Michelle Civalier

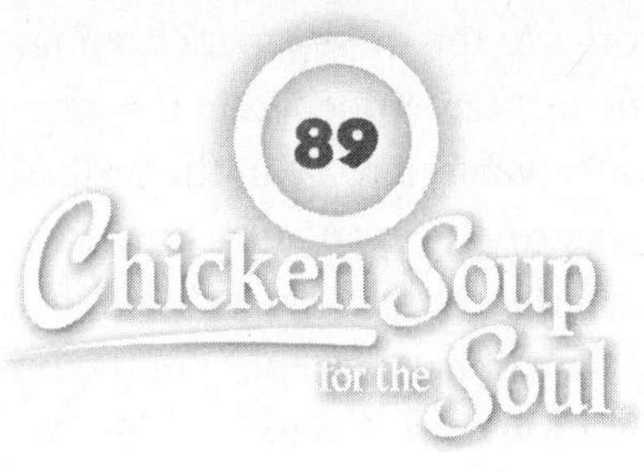

A Nurse with the Best Medicine

And in the sweetness of friendship let there be laughter and the sharing of pleasures. For in the dew of little things the heart finds its morning and is refreshed.
~*Kahlil Gibran*

It started nearly twenty years ago.

I would start coughing as soon as I lay down. Inconvenient and annoying, but not a huge deal. The professionals suggested it might be some mild type of asthma I'd just have to learn to live with. I did.

Then one fall, I went on a weekend retreat with several girlfriends at a cozy family cabin. One of these friends, Marci, was a long-time nurse and nursing instructor. Since three of us were sharing a bedroom, I crawled into my sleeping bag and warned the other two about my persistent cough.

Marci took on a most somber tone. "Oh," she said. "You have Chronic Nocturnal Positional Paroxysmal Bechesthesis."

My inner drama queen immediately took the spotlight. This sounded serious! How much time did I have left? Months? Days? Should I quit my job, put my affairs in order? No matter what, I would be brave.

"Really?" I managed to gasp. "What's that?"

"It means you cough when you lie down," Marci said.

The other friend, Lisa, let out a snort heard in Toronto and the two of them started chortling so hard they could hardly breathe. They rolled off their beds, which in turn got me laughing so hard I started a coughing fit that lasted long into the night. Which, in turn, made them howl even harder.

Although Marci made up the diagnosis, she provided the best medicine of all. I still get a boost of immunity-building endorphins whenever I recall that night we laughed so hard we all lost our breath.

~Terrie Todd

The Little Ways

We are each made for goodness, love and compassion. Our lives are transformed as much as the world is, when we live with these truths.

~Desmond Tutu

When you are a young active person with a clean bill of health, you never really expect to be hospitalized for two weeks. And you certainly never expect you will like it.

I was put in the hospital after I learned I had flesh-eating bacteria. I had been in a motorcycle accident a week prior and after getting twenty-six stitches I thought it was normal for my thigh to be sore, swollen and oozing blood. I was eighteen and didn't have any experience with serious injuries, so I didn't realize that the black spots around the stitches weren't normal.

I went to the hospital to get more gauze. It didn't take the nurse long to realize something was wrong. I was transferred to a bigger hospital and then into surgery that night. The surgeon cut a large chunk of my thigh right down to the muscle. I didn't know how deep it was for a few days because it had a huge bandage and a VAC machine.

I was on all sorts of painkillers and antibiotics, and I didn't know too much about what was going on for quite some time. I had to have a second surgery, but I still didn't know why. At that point, a few thoughts had entered my mind about possibly losing my leg, but the staff was all so positive around me, I didn't think about it too much.

My surgeon had encouraged me to go walking so I wouldn't lose my strength, and I didn't want to disobey him, so I walked a couple of times a day. During one walk late in the evening, I saw my surgeon sitting at the desk talking to another doctor. He gave me a big smile, so I stopped to talk to him. Since none of the nurses told me what was going on, I figured it would be a good time to ask him.

"You have necrotizing fasciitis," he said. From his tone, I could tell he figured I wouldn't understand his medical terminology.

"What does that mean?" I asked.

He chuckled, but then with a more serious look, said, "It means you're lucky that your wound was an open wound." I didn't understand, but didn't want to bother him with any other questions, so I continued my walk.

After almost a week at that hospital, I got transferred back to the little hospital where I had gone to get more gauze.

The nurses there weren't nearly as busy as the ones in the city and so they had more time to stay and chat. Right away, one of them commented on how lucky I was to have learned about the infection when I did. It probably wasn't good for me to know, but I couldn't resist asking her what would have happened if I'd found out later.

"You could have lost your leg," she said, "or worse."

Most of the time, I really did enjoy the hospital. I was the only young person there, so the nurses gave me special attention. On top of that, members from my church made multiple visits to see me and I got to sleep all the time.

The bad times usually happened when nobody was around and I couldn't sleep. I would be alone with the thoughts of how I could have died, and the irrational thoughts of how the antibiotics wouldn't work and my leg would be chopped off.

One night, when most of the patients were sleeping, I couldn't. My leg was sore, hot and puffy and I was on my cell phone looking up stuff about necrotizing fasciitis. I knew it wasn't a good idea, but I did it anyway. The more I read, the more certain I became that the bacteria would never go away and I would lose my leg. It was illogical, but in my defense I was drugged up and had a big chunk of my leg missing.

I got out of bed, trying to hold back my tears, and walked to the nurse's desk. I was going to ask if I could have something to help me sleep, but when the first nurse saw me she just gave me a hug and asked what was wrong.

"I'm scared," I said quietly. She held me as I cried. I told her what I was thinking about and she listened. Then she made me a banana split and invited me to sit at the desk with the nurses there. One of them talked to me about University, where I was starting my first year in the fall. It wasn't something I really wanted to focus on right then, but I stopped crying eventually, and ended up going to bed with a smile. Nobody had said anything in particular that calmed me down, or solved the problem, but those two nurses treated me with such kindness and love, it made me forget for a while why I was so upset.

It took four rounds of antibiotics, a month with the VAC machine, and lots and lots of waiting for my leg to heal, but it did. If it hadn't, I know there would've been nurses who held my hand through it.

I have quite a large scar on my leg and I love it. It reminds me of the goodness in people. No, it wasn't anything big; everyone at the hospital was there because it was their job to be there. In little ways though, they went above and beyond. That extra made a huge difference to this dumb kid who went looking for ways to scare herself.

~Emily Linegar

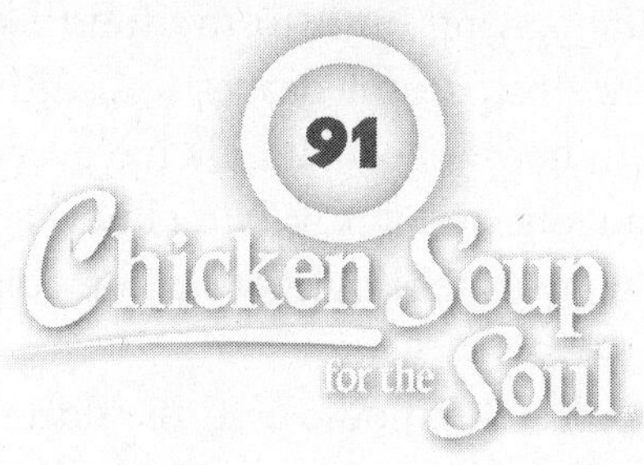

Sharing Hope

All it takes is one bloom of hope to make a spiritual garden.
~Terri Guillemets

"What was this little guy's birth weight?" It was a simple question, but it caught me off guard. I froze, unable to speak as my tears welled up.

Wondering why I didn't answer, with one hand safeguarding my baby on the scale, the nurse turned to face me. The bewildered expression on her beautiful face made me feel even more awkward and afraid.

A tear ran down my cheek as disturbing thoughts raced through my mind. "She's going to think I'm crazy. How do I explain? What mother doesn't know her own baby's birth weight?"

The truth was, I didn't know.

I wiped my cheek as every instinct within screamed at me to grab my baby and run. Instead, I stood there quivering and stared at this poor confused nurse.

She tried to comfort me, pleading in her gentle voice. "I'm so sorry. It's fine if you don't remember how much he weighed. Please don't be upset."

"It's not just that. It's… it's… everything," I cried. "I can't remember a single thing!"

That was a true statement.

Three weeks after giving birth to my fourth child, I was diagnosed with a severe postpartum depression. Although it came on instantly the moment he was born, it took me over a month to get up the courage to tell anyone about it. When I knew I couldn't go on any longer, I confided in my gynecologist, who immediately placed me in the care of a psychiatrist.

I was hospitalized within hours, and the doctor decided electroconvulsive therapy (ECT) would be the best treatment considering the seriousness of my condition. After two weeks of treatments in the hospital and several more as an outpatient, my short-term memory was seriously affected. I couldn't remember my stay in the hospital, nor could I remember most events that took place several months prior to the therapy. I would run into friends and not recognize them. I didn't remember events the rest of the family talked about. I was embarrassed and ashamed, my self-confidence completely destroyed.

Now, standing in the exam room during my baby son's four-month check-up, I was uncomfortable to say the least. I didn't want to tell the nurse why I couldn't remember his birth weight, nor did I want her to think I cared so little about him that I didn't even know the answer to such an important question. Still, I shied away from explaining the reason for my hesitation because of the stigma sometimes associated with mental illness.

Realizing I'd most likely be faced with the same situation as soon as the pediatrician came into the room, I decided to tell her the truth. She seemed nice, but I seriously doubted she'd understand.

"I don't usually share this, but the reason I'm having such a difficult time trying to remember things is because I've had shock therapy for postpartum depression." Whew, I said it.

With a look of understanding and compassion on her face she said, "I know how you feel, hon."

"Sure she does," I thought sarcastically, wallowing in self-pity.

Before I could reply, she stunned me with, "I've been where you are right now. Three years ago, after my son was born, I suffered from postpartum depression and had to undergo shock therapy, too. Believe me, things do get better."

I don't know if it was because I had finally met someone who actually understood what I was going through or because she told me that things would get better; but, whatever the reason, tears of relief flowed.

As she finished weighing and measuring my son, she continued, "I've never told any of my coworkers, let alone perfect strangers. Mental illness, especially any involving hospitalization and electroconvulsive therapy, is subject to preconceived notions by those who are unfamiliar with how difficult it can be. I figure it's better to keep it to myself. I had to share with you because you looked so sad, and I wanted you to know that I got through it, and you will, too.

"I'll write down Darren's current weight and length so you'll have it handy," she said with a wink.

As she was handing me the small piece of paper, the doctor walked in and greeted us with a smile, putting an end to our conversation.

Fortunately he didn't ask any questions during the exam that put me in an uncomfortable position. I breathed a sigh of relief as I bundled up my baby boy and headed home.

Later that evening as I was organizing the diaper bag and putting things away, I pulled out the slip of paper the nurse had given me with the baby's information on it. I smiled when I noticed that she had drawn a happy smile next to her phone number and the words, "If you ever need to talk, give me a call."

I will forever be grateful to this sweet nurse who not only looked out for the wellbeing of her little patient, but for his mother as well. And she was absolutely right — things did get better, largely in part to a special nurse who stepped out of her comfort zone to offer hope.

~Connie Kaseweter Pullen

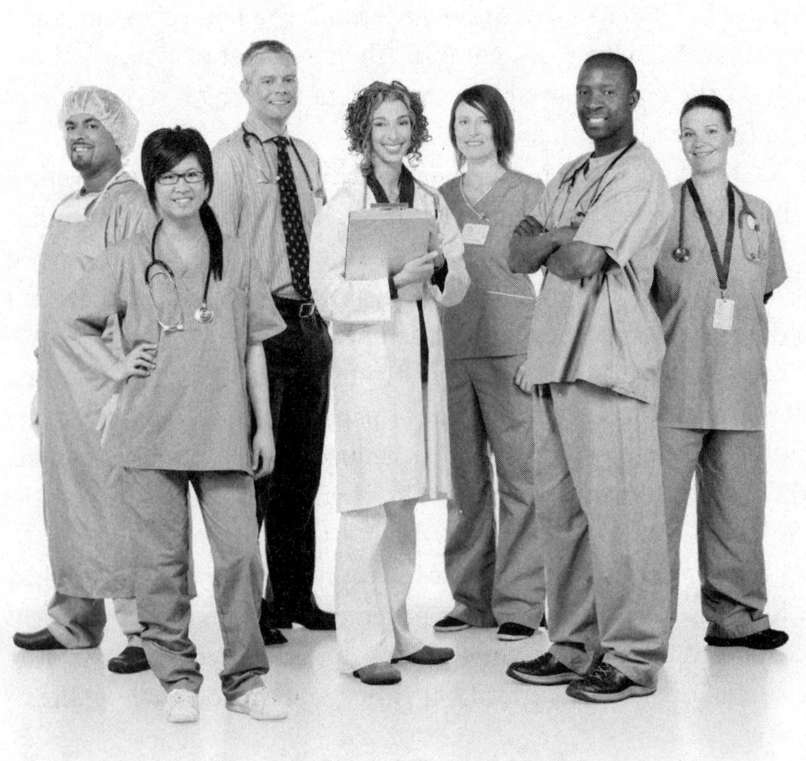

Inspiration for Nurses

Thank You

As we express our gratitude, we must never forget that the highest appreciation is not to utter words, but to live by them.

~John F. Kennedy

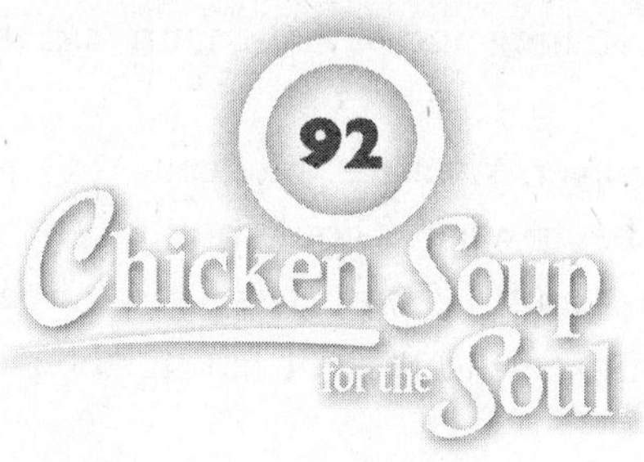

You Were My Arms

Gratitude is the memory of the heart.
~Italian Proverb

It was a heartbreaking call. Our grandson, David, was in the hospital, his cancer advanced. He needed an emergency procedure.

"Oh, Mom." My daughter was nearly weeping.

I'd already been weeping for her all day. I had to remain strong. I'd been at the computer, finding emergency flights for David's siblings, plus transportation to airports and the distant hospital. Finally the last ticket was for our pastor, who was also our son-in-law's long-time friend. He could embrace Frank, give him a shoulder to cry on. He would get there in time. But who would be there for my Cheri?

My heart was breaking. It was not just a saying, I could feel it. What mother does not want to be with her daughter at a time like this to hold her? To comfort her. But I could not be there. I was thousands of miles away.

The call disconnected before I could offer love or prayers. Only tears. I waited and prayed into the silent night.

The phone rang again. "Oh, Mom, something went wrong." Then silence. Disconnected again.

"Oh, God. Please send someone to be my arms for my child."

And you were there. You held her. You wept with her and prayed with her. You told her what you saw, and what she needed to hear, that others were watching and saw the faith and the peace amid the pain.

You were my prayer. My arms. My tears.

Thank you for being where I could not be. Thank you for explaining all the machines and the processes, and for easing my daughter and son-in-law's impossible task of letting their son go to God as gently as possible.

Thank you for doing more than your job that night… for being an intercessor, a constant source of comfort. For holding her for me, letting your heart break with hers, yet being an accepting, believing, encouraging rock. Your compassion comforted a mom and her daughter at the same time across the country. You were God's conduit.

You say you are "just a nurse." But you raised the definition of nurse to a new level that night. You suffered with… acted in place of… substituted for her mom with full efficiency and tender compassion. You helped to get the phone so I could talk to my grandson and my daughter. I've never thanked you for all those things. But how could I?

I don't even know your full name. God and his angels do, and for you that was enough. Your willingness to step into the breach was truly a Godsend. The hours you spent beyond your shift, a treasure. You have glorified the calling.

So thank you, nurse.

Thank you for being this mother's heart.

Thank you for being my arms.

~Delores Christian Liesner

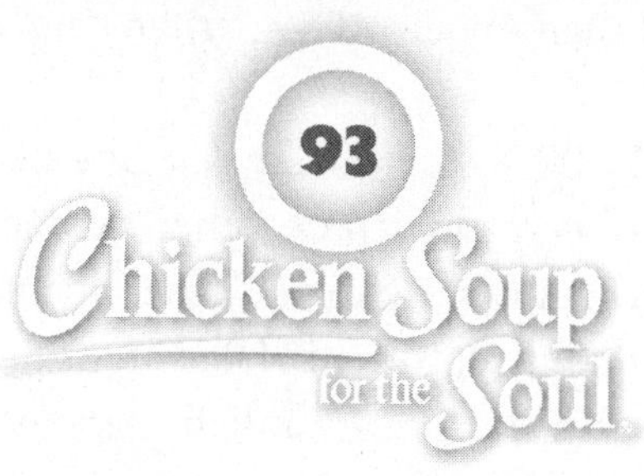

Nurse Carrie

The crisis of today is the joke of tomorrow.
~H. G. Wells

Turning twelve was a big deal for my niece, Haley. It was the age when my brother said she could get her ears pierced and start wearing make-up in public. Since this was clearly a milestone, I planned a trip to a day spa for a first make-up lesson and fun. We stopped for an early lunch first at a little steakhouse.

Three bites into her steak, Haley's face got bright red and she started slapping herself on the back of the neck. Understanding hit me just as suddenly. "Haley, are you choking?"

She nodded.

"Can you get any air at all?"

She shook her head.

I pulled her out of the booth and tried to do the Heimlich maneuver, but it didn't work.

I like to think I remained stoic in the face of crisis, that I calmly asked for assistance, but I'm pretty sure I started screaming for help like a crazy person. Because I was a crazy person at that moment. Crazy with fear and, for thirty of the longest seconds of my life, sure that my niece was going to die right in my arms.

I was hollering for help and for the hostess to call 911 and doing a weird half-praying, half-screaming thing that I am confident God understood… and then my Good Samaritan came.

Nurse Carrie.

It was barely 11:00 so there weren't many people in the restaurant. In fact, there were only nine other people in the restaurant then… and one of them was Nurse Carrie. She came running over, yelled that she was a nurse, turned Haley around, wrapped her arms around her torso, and did the Heimlich maneuver hard enough to yank Haley off her feet.

Twice.

And the steak came flying out.

The next few minutes were a blur of tears, hugs, and the manager fawning all over us like the whole choking issue was his fault. I managed to get Nurse Carrie's first name in all the commotion but then she faded into the background while I tried to calm down.

At which point Haley looked up at me fearfully and put things in true twelve-year-old perspective. "Did I look stupid?"

Man, I love that kid.

In any case, I've never seen Nurse Carrie again and the odds she will ever see this are really quite slim. But I think of her often and pray for her more.

God bless you, Nurse Carrie, wherever you are.

~Kimberly Yates

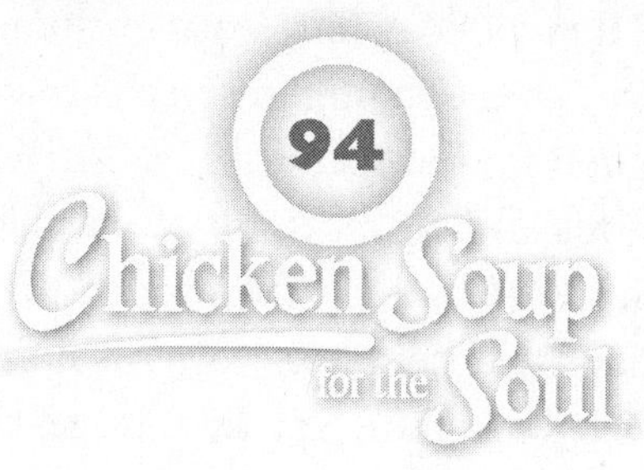

Heart to Heart Talk

Knowledge comes, but wisdom lingers.
~Alfred Lord Tennyson

After having two healthy children and handling earaches and colic, I thought I had motherhood down. Then our third child came into the world. Ashley was born with several life threatening heart complications. As our pediatrician examined her, his doctor-like grunts and groans struck fear in my heart. When he told me to call my husband and take our baby five hours north to see specialists, we left immediately.

We arrived late in the evening at the University Hospital where a group of cardiologists waited for us. After asking me a multitude of questions, they whisked my fragile daughter away to prep her for an emergency heart surgery. I began pacing in the waiting room when a kind-faced nurse named Alice approached me. She gently placed her hand on my shoulder, and then patiently proceeded to tell me everything that was happening with our baby and what to expect for the next few days. Her confidence and compassion helped calm my worried heart.

Watching my helpless infant struggle in pain and being unable to comfort her was hard to bear. The doctors were capable, the surgeons were skilled, but the nurses were the ones who held me together and gave my daughter the nurturing I couldn't.

After the operation, when the surgeons came for their regular rounds, they made it obvious Ashley wasn't responding well. She was covered in cords and wires leading to screens that revealed numbers that did not look good for her recovery. The surgeons recommended some medication, but all I could think of was how much I wanted to hold my baby in my arms. I felt she needed that as much as I did.

After the surgeons left the room, it was as if this astute nurse was reading my mind. "It will take some time to get the order in for the medication," Alice informed me. "In the meantime, let's try this."

Then she scooped Ashley up in one arm, and in one smooth movement used her other arm to wrap half a dozen leads and cords in a circular motion around my baby. Then she handed the bundle to me… cords, blanket, baby and all.

"Now, Mom," she addressed me, "cuddle and nurse her and let's watch those numbers stabilize on the monitor." Alice was right. We both watched as Ashley's numbers normalized. She was out of cardiac recovery and in a regular hospital room within hours. "Nothing like a mother's love to give a baby what she needs," Alice commented with a smile.

The caring nurse continued with her helpful insight and compassionate care while Ashley slowly recovered. As I was preparing to take her home, Alice walked me through the steps to care for my fragile post-operative newborn. When she finished her instructions, she sat down on the edge of the bed, looked me in the eye and said, "You have to be very careful not to create a cardiac cripple." Her sober tone caught me off guard.

Reading my expression, she went on to explain. "You are going to want to hover over her and keep her from doing things because you are worried that she is too fragile."

"That's exactly what I plan to do," I blurted. "I've just spent the last ten days watching this delicate baby cling to life and I have every intention of walking out of here and protecting her from anything and everything, even if it means her foot never touches the ground for as long as she lives!" I tried not to cry as her words of truth broke down my fearful exterior.

"I know," said the wise nurse. "I can see it in your face. As hard as it will be to resist the urge, you can't hover. You have to let her regulate herself so she won't grow up weak and helpless. She'll know what her limits are. Let her govern her own activity. With all she has to deal with for the rest of her life, she needs to feel as strong as possible."

Alice's words were profound. I have referred to that conversation more times than I can count in my daughter's life. That's why Ashley is a twenty-nine-year-old strong, confident, and capable young woman today.

~Linda Newton

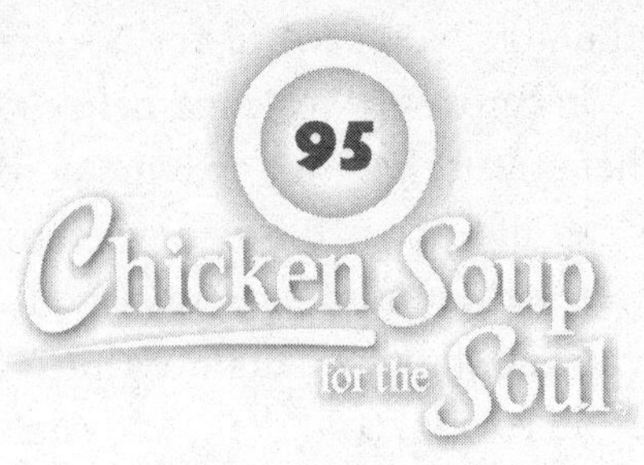

Payback

A teacher affects eternity; he can never tell where his influences stop.
~Henry Adams

By the time I reached fourth grade I was taller than everyone in my class. Truth be told, I was taller than every kid in the Epiphany Grammar School, and even my teacher my teacher, Miss Liston. Unfortunately my height far surpassed my coordination, agility, and scholastic aptitude. I became the class clown, and not by choice. I struggled with arithmetic, spelling and reading. Recess was even worse, when everyone ran around playing games and sports. Clumsy was my middle name.

Each afternoon Miss Liston finished the day by reading to the class for fifteen minutes. I was relieved to see the end of another day's string of embarrassments and would lose myself in her voice and the story, usually a chapter book such as *Danny, The Champion of the World*. During those quiet minutes I watched her read effortlessly, magically, as though she recognized every word, a talent I yearned to be mine. If I could read with such ease I could find my way to happier places and times. I could grow up like my father, who seemed to spend the end of every evening behind the cover of his beloved books. Miss Liston apparently took notice of my rapt attention. I don't remember how she took me under her wing but by the time I moved on to fifth grade I was reading at an eighth-grade level. My self-image, self-esteem, and life path were altered forever.

When asked, "What do you want to be when you grow up?" I had an absolutely certain response: "I want to read." I was still unaware that Professional Reader was not a viable career path. By my senior year of high school that goal had morphed into becoming a journalist.

During my junior year of college I dropped out. I found a job as a newspaper reporter and discovered that while I had the diligence and desire to be a journalist, I had neither the education nor the talent to succeed. Five years of struggling to write one good sentence were enough. I quit writing. But I couldn't quit eating or pay my rent with my good looks. I quickly found a job as an operating room orderly at a local hospital. I was fascinated by the science, inter-personal connectivity, and outright compassion that seemed to enable patients to heal.

A friendly, insightful nursing school instructor who watched me transport frightened patients to the OR took me aside one day and suggested that I consider becoming a registered nurse. At that time, male RNs were rare. It took another year for me to make the leap.

I found nursing school to be far easier than most of my classmates. I could read, write term papers and patient care plans, and study with effortlessness and pleasure.

One early spring evening during my first year as an emergency room nurse, an ambulance brought an elderly woman in who'd apparently suffered a stroke. She was secured on the stretcher and covered with several sheets and a blanket. As I approached, the paramedic began his report. "We have a seventy-eight-year-old woman, Agnes Liston, found at home by neighbors…" I didn't hear the rest. I quickly, gently folded back the sheet to better see Miss Liston's ancient, now drooping face. Silently, I smiled at her a long moment until she could focus through her fright. "Hello, Miss Liston. It's me, Tommy Schwarz. Do you remember me?" I asked softly. She stared back and her facial muscles twitched. "I'll take that as a 'Yes'."

I learned that as a life-long spinster, she'd outlived family and friends. No one came to visit her while she was hospitalized except me. For the next three days I sat at her bedside reading to her. She was unable to communicate her boredom or appreciation. I like to think she recognized every word. It looked like she felt comforted. I felt privileged to give back in a direct and personal way to someone who had loved and helped me so much.

~Thom Schwarz

My Soldier

I may be compelled to face danger, but never fear it,
and while our soldiers can stand and fight,
I can stand and feed and nurse them.
~Clara Barton

While in nursing school I always pictured myself working in the ER. I loved the fast-paced environment and the quick decision-making. To my surprise, I landed on the Oncology/Palliative Care unit at the VA Hospital. There could not have been a place more opposite of where I had pictured myself. Instead of fast-paced, I was in an area that was quiet and slow, one of impending closure.

For many of our veterans this is the last step, the last battle they will fight. There is no greater reward than to be with someone as they transition from this life to the next.

I met one quiet hero on an evening shift. He had suffered greatly throughout his life. Being a gay man in the military in the 1960s and 1970s was a hard road to travel. He developed HIV in the 1980s and had expected he would die from that disease, but surprisingly that was not the case. Instead he developed cancer.

When I first met him he came strolling down the hallway with his walker. He was a rather large man who had led a very sedentary lifestyle. Just getting around his home stressed him. We spent hours visiting throughout his stays. He shared his life and I shared mine.

We laughed at the funny times and cried together during the low ones.

One night we were sharing our "bucket lists." I told him the things I hoped to do one day, but said I was waiting until the time was right. Sitting in his darkened room he shared how he had done the same thing. Unfortunately, when he finally felt the time was right, he had cancer and was unable to do all that he had waited for.

"Don't wait," he told me. "Get out there and do the things you want to do."

While I sat talking and watching this once-strong solider crying because of what he had lost, I decided to start living my life at that moment as if it were my last.

The next summer I skydived, raced cars, went whitewater rafting, and ran my first half marathon. I came back after each activity and shared my adventure with him. He was living through me. After I ran my first half marathon, we talked about the importance of exercise, healthy lifestyles, and getting out there doing whatever you could do.

I began running in various races for charities. After each one, I shared with him the highlights, the training before, the cramps during, and running in the rain and in the heat.

After every race he got more excited until one night he told me, "I want to do a race with you."

I loved the idea but knew realistically that would never happen. How could an overweight, sedentary man dying from cancer ever be able to do a 5K?

Over the next year I watched in awe and admiration as he transformed himself. He started by doing one lap around the unit, slowly taking each step with his walker. Soon he was doing several laps. He lost weight and became more active. Each time he was admitted, I could see his spirits increasing. He was happy again, smiling and encouraged. He had a new goal and couldn't wait to achieve it. At home, he had finally worked up to walking a mile, always with his walker. He was never going to be fast, but his determination was inspiring.

It was fall when we decided to participate in the upcoming breast cancer walk the next spring. I had lost my mother to breast cancer when she was fifty-four years old and had shared with him how important breast cancer research and awareness was to me.

"Let's do the breast cancer walk in memory of your mom," he insisted.

Over the next several months we planned our outfits, our pace, and even our snacks. He would bake his wonderful cookies. His mom became involved in the excitement and the planning, as did his son. We worked so hard on our plans that we actually looked forward to his hospital stays so we could continue with our strategizing!

He designed the T-shirt we would wear, one that represented past and present warriors fighting cancers of all types.

Everything was lining up just perfectly for our walk in April. That was until March, when my soldier took a turn for the worse. Life changes on a dime and this was never more evident to me as I watched my friend slowly slipping away. The week before the race he was admitted for his last time. His hard battle was nearing its end.

One day his son told me they were taking him off the ventilator. I just couldn't believe it. It wasn't fair! His son asked me to come and say goodbye and through tears I told him I just couldn't do it.

"I understand," he said. "Just know how important you were to Dad and how happy you made him these past months." He hugged me, then cried as he walked away.

I struggled for the next few minutes and finally decided I had to say goodbye. This man had done so much to change who I was. I had to see him off as I had done with so many other veterans. I ran down the two flights of stairs, down the hall and as I approached his room, I heard the doctor pronounce the time of death. I was too late. I had missed my chance to say goodbye.

His mom came out and told me he had gone peacefully. We hugged and cried. There were no words to share. Our soldier fought the battle hard but wasn't able to win this war. Cancer once again was the victor.

At work the following Friday, the night before the race, I was surprised to see my soldier's mom and son come to the floor.

"We came to do the race with you," they said in unison.

Astonished, I shook my head and admitted, "Without him I lost my desire to compete."

"Oh no," the son said. "Remember what Dad said. 'Get out there now and do the things you want to do.'"

He reached into a bag and pulled out the shirts his dad had designed and made for us to wear. "We will walk in memory of your mom as planned, and now in memory of Dad."

~Jacqueline K. Brumley

The Extra Mile

Grief can be the garden of compassion. If you keep your heart open through everything, your pain can become your greatest ally in your life's search for love and wisdom.
~Rumi

Self-doubt knotted my stomach as I approached the Alzheimer's assisted-living facility. I signed in at the desk and pinned the Evergreen Place guest badge onto my jacket. Then I entered the residential area and started to search.

The main room appeared empty. On second glance, however, I spotted the salt-and-pepper hair of one woman sitting by herself, head down, dozing on the couch.

"Mom? Mom, it's time to eat lunch." I lowered myself beside her and wrapped one arm around her shoulders. "Wake up, Mom. It's me."

Her eyes fluttered open. "Who?"

"Beth. Your daughter." The one you haven't known for years, I thought. The one who doesn't come around as often as she ought to.

I stood to face her, embraced her in a bear hug, and attempted to hoist her up. Two times I tried and failed. I wondered if she had forgotten how to stand. Finally, on the third attempt, she rose. But when I let go with one arm to sling my purse over my shoulder, she collapsed onto the couch, eyes wide with terror. Not knowing what to do, I paused until Halley, one of the young activity leaders, arrived.

"Hey five-foot-two eyes of blue." Flashing a warm smile, Halley bent down to look into Mom's eyes. "I came looking for you."

Mom lifted her neck enough to see who was speaking to her while Halley expertly boosted Mom to her feet.

"It's good to see you," said Halley as she winked at me.

I wrapped one hand around Mom's waist. Together we took slow steps down the short hall. We passed tiny alcoves painted with color. The pretend post office. The library. The beauty shop. The law office. With her head bent down, Mom saw none of it.

When we reached the dining room, I maneuvered Mom to her place. Her sweet tea, a bowl of grapes, and some minestrone soup were waiting. The nurses had even remembered her straw.

"Mom, you need to sit down." I wheeled a chair up behind her, helped her plop down into it, and scooted her up to the table. From behind the kitchen's serving counter, Mom's favorite nurse nodded and sent me a reassuring grin. Then I started to feed Mom.

Dad had warned me. "She can't feed herself anymore. You'll have to touch the spoon to her lips and hope she opens. She'll chew each bite twenty times, close her eyes, and fall asleep. Or, she'll push herself up from the table and leave."

Eighteen residents sat and fed themselves, unable to talk with one another. Except for the nurses, Mom and I were the only ones who attempted conversation even though Mom could no longer put together a coherent sentence.

"Someone else has come to lunch. Blanche is waving at you, Mom."

Sitting diagonally across from us, the resident stared. "What's wrong with her?" she blurted out as she pointed to my mom. I chose to ignore her question, not wanting to attempt to explain that early-onset Alzheimer's had begun to ravage Mom's mind twelve years ago. Now, at age seventy-one, there wasn't much of it left. The first-grade teacher who had lovingly instructed others could no longer be taught.

Two nurses approached with Mom's main course. "Ms. Ellen, you're sliding down again. Do you need help?" The nurses positioned themselves on either side of Mom and lifted her to a better sitting position. "There you go, Ms. Ellen. Good job."

I was probably doing everything wrong. By gently stepping in to assist when necessary, however, the nurses encouraged me without words. They even slipped a glass of tea, a cup of chicken noodle soup, and a salad in front of me, saying, "This is for you." I wasn't sure they were supposed to do that but, hungry, I accepted.

Two hours later, Mom finally finished her lunch. Knowing what she probably needed, I walked her over to a couple of nurses and timidly said, "I think my mom has to use the restroom."

"Let us help you." Relief washed over me, because Dad had told me it could get ugly. And, it did.

Not understanding what was happening when the nurses tried to assist her, Mom pushed them away. She kicked them. She swore. Despite Mom's outburst, the nurses skillfully cleaned her, changed her, and somehow continued to speak kind words to her. The moment they finished, the strangest thing happened. Mom grabbed the hands of one nurse, started to sing, "Doo, de doo, de doo," and swiveled her hips. The nurse danced along with her.

Afterwards, because she couldn't sit still and seldom napped, I decided to walk with Mom. We meandered through the hallways of the other buildings' wings. Sometimes Mom's face contorted. She pointed to things that weren't there. Unable to express what she was feeling, she uttered four-letter words she never used to speak.

"Everything is okay, Mom." Entering into her world, I tried to reassure her. Most of the time it worked, but I was exhausted. I wondered how Dad did this for ten hours every day and how the nurses covered for him during the time he wasn't with her.

When we walked through the blue nursing wing, however, I finally understood. Patients lay on hospital beds around the nurse's station or in their tiny rooms. I heard no laughter, saw no movement, observed little life. This was what Dad was trying to keep Mom from.

The Evergreen Place nurses had told Dad this was where Mom technically needed to be now. She was past the assisted-living care they normally provided. They shouldn't have to feed her breakfast. Or endure her fear-induced fight to help her use the bathroom, bathe, dress, or get ready for bed. They'd chosen to go the extra mile, though. For my mom's sake. And for my dad's.

After two hours of walking, Mom and I wandered back to Evergreen Place. Back to the nurses who engaged the residents in conversation, who painted their patients' nails, who honored them with respect they'd never remember. Back to another two-hour feeding. Back to Mom's small room where nurses had thoughtfully laid out her nightgown, placed pads on her bed, and turned down her bedcovers.

Needing to return home to my husband and two young children, I escorted Mom toward Catherine, a nursing assistant with beautiful black braids.

"Catherine, I need to go now. Could you help my mom?" I didn't want to ask. Dad had told me about Mom's fear of getting ready for bed. About the flailing, the hitting, the cursing.

"Of course."

Of course? When she knew the battle she'd soon be facing?

Yes, of course, because even though the lady the nurses cared for was only a fragment of who she used to be, they knew none of this was her fault. They honored and loved her anyway.

Catherine took Mom's hands. "Ms. Ellen, we'll be just fine, won't we?" In response, once again Mom swung her hips and started to dance.

My heart, filled with gratitude for those who cared for Mom, danced along with them.

~Beth Saadati

You Are Only Blind If You Refuse to See

The only real voyage of discovery consists not in seeking new landscapes but in having new eyes.
~Marcel Proust

"Miss Flora," I said one day in my calmest voice as a rat meandered past the table. "Did you know you have rats?"

"Darn! I thought so. I'll get me some poison and put it down," she said. Subject closed; no big deal.

When I moved to Florida, I had no idea how different my life would be. I had been excited about relocating but did not anticipate feeling like such a stranger in a strange land. As a home health nurse, I quickly found myself looking at life from the other side as I leapt feet first into my new job.

Miss Flora was an elderly diabetic whom I visited daily for insulin injections. Every day, as I administered her medication, she gave me a good dose of reality in return. Having been blind for a number of years and living with a sister who was also blind, her reality was fixed in her memory. It fell to me to tread that fine line between how things really were and how she remembered them to be.

She spoke with fondness of the house she lived in, hand-built by her daddy, but unknown to her, in a sad state of disrepair. She did not see the fine piles of sawdust under each table leg where termites slowly had their way, the regular parade of cockroaches, or the road map of cracks in the plaster.

"Miss Flora," I said, when I arrived a few days later. "There's a dead rat on your floor."

"Okay, baby," she said, calm as ever. "Just put a paper towel in my hand and guide it down to it so I can pick it up."

Now, I am not a fan of rodents, dead or alive, but what kind of person lets a little, elderly blind lady pick up a dead rat?

"Don't worry," I said. I put a glove on and picked it up myself. The tail felt weird and rubbery as I held it at arm's length, and I prayed that it was truly dead. Gingerly holding that nasty rat the size of a small cat, I gratefully dropped it into the trash. It was a job I repeated several more times over the ensuing weeks.

"Where do you live?" she asked me one day. When I told her, she replied matter-of-factly, "When I was young and living here, colored people weren't allowed in that neighborhood after the sun went down."

"Excuse me?" I said, at a loss for words.

"Sure," she said. "We had a lot of rules about where we could go, where we had to live. We even had our own beach over on the bay. Never did see the ocean."

"You live five miles from the Gulf of Mexico, and you've never seen it?" I asked, stunned.

"No colored people allowed," she repeated. I was speechless. Now of course, she was unable to see anything, so the experience of seeing the ocean was an opportunity lost forever. I began to see Miss Flora with new eyes.

Over time, I learned a number of things about her. She was once a prize-winning Lindy dancer and lived in New York City during the days of the Cotton Club. She knew important people in the early days of NBC. She had a wicked sense of humor. She lived large during a time when many people tended to be quite small-minded. This blind lady truly opened my eyes.

Just before my first baby was born, Miss Flora presented me with a small package in a mailing wrapper. "Got something for that baby of yours," she said shyly.

I was caught completely unaware, both touched and dismayed, as I knew a gift for me was something she could ill afford. Hesitant to rob her of the joy of the moment, I did not voice my concern for the cost. While she waited expectantly, I tore open the package. I pulled out two tiny sleepers, one pink, one purple, and turned to her in gratitude. I wondered how she had managed to make a phone call all alone and place an order. I marveled at how a woman who grew up in a rigidly segregated society could find herself giving a gift to a white baby she would never see. I thought about what a miracle it was that a blind woman who had seen so much ugliness could have such generosity in her heart.

I said, "Thank you. It's exactly what I needed." She smiled broadly.

When my son was born, he wore that pink sleeper right along with the purple one, and when he outgrew it, I stored it away with all the other outfits that had special meaning to me.

Miss Flora's funeral took place at a small Baptist church in a neighborhood where few people ventured alone. I took both children, my daughter just an infant, my son a toddler, to witness the going home of a very fine lady.

Recently, my twenty-year-old son asked, "Hey Mom, remember when we went to Miss Flora's funeral? I think about her sometimes, don't you?"

He couldn't have been more than three at the time. "Yes," I said. "I think about her a lot.

Though she was blind, she taught us to see that we find special people in all sorts of places, often where we least expect it."

~Sharon Stoika-Smay

Grace

I do not at all understand the mystery of grace — only that it meets us where we are but does not leave us where it found us.
~Anne Lamott

"I should be studying for mid-terms," I thought, "not lying here in bed." But my mystery illness forced me to return home from college mid-semester, and now I had to wait for a referral to a specialist, one who was booked until the end of the month.

I had been so positive about getting answers for my muscle weakness, but I woke up with my emotions just as heavy as my body. I started doubting the hope I was holding on to. At this point, I had been lying in bed for two months with no improvement.

I was falling in and out of sleep when I heard a knock at the door. It was my physical therapist. She took one look at me and said, "Skipping P.T. today?" I was so weak I couldn't respond. She asked me to lift my head. I couldn't. She seemed confused as to why I had gotten so much worse. We skipped that day and she went home.

I tried rolling to my side, but I couldn't do it. I felt so helpless. I just stayed there in bed with my eyes closed, wanting to escape from reality.

A few hours later, there was knock at the door again. It was a nurse. After I had fainted from exhaustion at the doctor's office a month prior, he decided I was too weak to leave my house, so he ordered in-home care. But it was a Friday night. Nurses never came this late.

My mom walked the nurse upstairs to my bedroom. She looked very concerned.

"Hi, Alyssa, I'm Grace," she said. "I saw your blood work, and your numbers are all over the place. We need to get you into a hospital soon."

"We've been trying to get to a specialist so she can be referred to a different hospital, but she's been stuck on a wait list," my mom explained.

"You know what?" Grace said. "My brother worked at USC Medical Center. I'll get you an appointment there first thing Monday morning."

Up until this point, doctors had been telling me that I was stressed and just needed rest, or that something was so wrong that life as I knew it would never be the same. What I needed was someone to acknowledge that I was living in a very dark place, and to shine some light into my situation. Thank God for Grace.

Saturday morning, I woke up to the sound of my dad and brothers coming home from a baseball game. My dad came right up to see me. "How are you feeling?"

I just shook my head.

"You want to get up and try to walk around?" I just closed my eyes. He had no idea how weak and exhausted my body was. There was no way I could walk.

My brother Frankie came up to talk to my dad. I focused in on their conversation. It felt good to have life around me.

As they talked, I turned back inward and realized it was becoming more and more difficult to breathe. I tried not to panic or exert too much energy as I fought for even the smallest breath.

"Can't breathe." I could barely get the words.

I tried again, using every ounce of energy I had. "Can't breathe." I had my dad's attention now. "Take me to USC."

With my mom on one side and my dad on the other, they walked me down the stairs and into the front seat of our Suburban. My dad sped all the way as I focused on inhaling and exhaling. Finally, we arrived at USC Medical Center. Because of Grace, my name was in their system and I was approved to be checked in and seen by their doctors.

The doctors immediately diagnosed me with the muscle disease called myasthenia gravis. They explained that I was in the process of having a myasthenic crisis, and a few days later, discovered a cancerous tumor near my heart.

They found all of this and more. They not only diagnosed me accurately, but they treated me with excellence. Medications, intubations, chemotherapy, radiation, and surgeries were all a part of my healing process. It was a long journey, but I can now breathe, walk, and talk on my own, living a full life. I even picked up where I left off in school and completed my master's degree.

I found out later that Grace was off work that night when she came to my house. She was in her car skimming through her paperwork when she came across my file and saw how serious my blood work results looked. She felt compelled to see me immediately.

Without Grace coming to my house that day, I don't know what would have happened to me. She was an intuitive nurse who went above and beyond.

She gave me grace in human form.

~Alyssa Annunziato

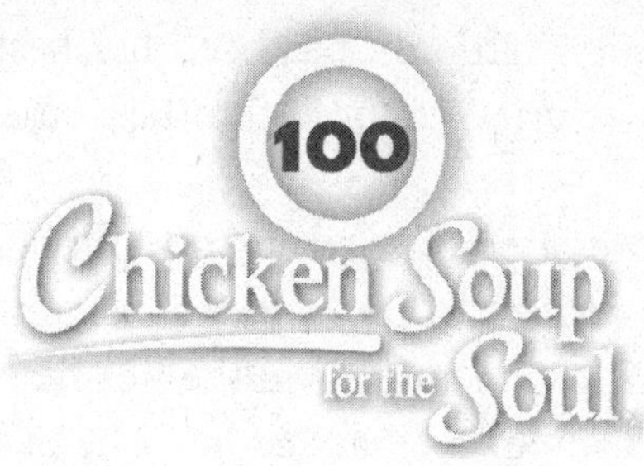

Breaking the Rules

I follow three rules: Do the right thing, do the best you can, and always show people you care.
~Lou Holtz

My mother was diagnosed with terminal cancer long before hospitals in our part of the country had heard of "pet therapy" for patients. So when I asked at the nurse's station if it would be possible for me to bring Little Bit, Mother's beloved Chihuahua, to visit her hospital room, I received the expected answer.

"A dog in the hospital? Certainly not!"

"But she's a tiny dog," I pleaded. "Only seven pounds."

"Doesn't matter," the charge nurse replied, shaking her head. "This hospital prides itself on cleanliness. And dogs are certainly not clean."

"How about if I give her a bath before we come?"

Again, the nurse shook her head. "It's not just that. The patients on this floor are very ill, as you know. They require peace and quiet. We can't have dogs barking."

"Little Bit isn't much of a barker." I forced a smile. "Unless there's a cat around. And I'm betting you don't allow cats here either."

"Nope."

I felt tears well up and tried to swallow them back. "My mother has been a widow for almost ten years," I said, trying to keep my voice from trembling. "Little Bit has been her best friend ever since my dad died. They're grieving for each other. Surely you can understand that."

The nurse's expression softened and she put her hand on my arm. "I do understand and I wish I could say yes. Really I do. But rules are rules. And the rules say no animals in the hospital."

I offered a weak smile and thanked her. Then I turned and walked toward the wall of elevators, knowing there was only one solution. If I couldn't march Little Bit into the hospital at the end of her leash, I'd smuggle her in. And I knew just how to do it.

But first, as promised, I would bathe her. No easy task with a dog who hated water, even one who only weighed seven pounds. I lathered and rinsed Little Bit twice and then rubbed her dry with a fluffy towel, hoping that once the wet dog smell went away she'd be fragrant as a flower. Or at least not as stinky as before I wrestled her into the tub.

Then I called my brother-in-law Tim.

He and my sister were going to pick me up on their way to the hospital the next day. "Wear your biggest, loosest coat," I told him.

"Why? It's not supposed to be cold."

I explained my plan.

"Of course I'll do it," he said. "But I sure hope they don't call the police on us."

In the hospital parking lot the next day, Tim unzipped his jacket and slipped Little Bit inside. "Be still and be quiet," he told her, "because you're going to love where we're going." As though she understood every word he was saying, Little Bit settled in on the right side of Tim's chest. Tim shoved his hand into his pocket so he could support her weight in the crook of his elbow and zipped up the jacket.

Then into the lobby, up the elevator and past the nurse's station we went.

I waved at the charge nurse who was talking on the phone and paid us little mind. As luck would have it, Mother was alone in her room. She looked awful, even paler and thinner and weaker than the day before. I leaned over the bedrail and kissed her crepe-paper cheek. "We've brought you a surprise," I whispered.

"Did you?" Her smile was half-hearted.

But there was nothing half-hearted in what happened when Tim unzipped his jacket. Little Bit sprang into Mother's arms and covered her face with kisses. Tears and giggles and wags and wiggles and the happiest dog whimpering filled that bleak hospital room. Before I could suggest that Mother slip Little Bit under the covers, there was a quick rap on the door and in walked Ashley, Mother's favorite nurse. She was kind, gentle and seldom in a hurry. But she was also a consummate professional who knew all the hospital rules.

What would she do about Little Bit?

Ashley's eyes grew wide when she saw the tiny black dog cradled in Mother's arms. "Well… who do we have here?"

In a voice stronger than I'd heard her use in days, Mother answered. "I bet you can guess."

Ashley crossed the room and reached out to stroke Little Bit between the ears. "I've heard all about you," she said softly. "I'm glad you came to visit." Little Bit wagged and wiggled some more. "But we have to keep this a secret because dogs aren't allowed in the hospital. So I'm going to put a note on the door saying you're having private family time."

"Thank you," I said, not even trying to swallow back tears.

Mother and Little Bit snuggled for almost half an hour, until Ashley slipped back into the room. "Shift change," she said. "Better get you-know-who out of here." She handed me a slip of paper. "Here's my work schedule for next week. In case you know someone who'd like to visit while I'm on duty."

I gave her a quick hug as Tim tucked Little Bit into his jacket.

I whispered a prayer of gratitude for nurses who understand that sometimes, the best rule is to break one.

~Jennie Ivey

Profound Words

I have just three things to teach: simplicity, patience, compassion. These three are your greatest treasures.
~Lao Tzu

In the 1980s, I took a part-time weekend job as a hospice nurse, visiting terminally ill patients in their homes. After a month of on-the-job orientation, I was on my own. My first solo visit was to a young man dying of AIDS. His chart indicated he had been a hospice patient for only a short time and was near death. As I drove to his house I wondered what I could do for him. I wondered about his pre-AIDS life. Had he gone to college? What kind of work had he done? Had he been successful? Did his family disown him when he was diagnosed with this dread disease? AIDS in the 1980s. So many fears. So much still to learn.

As I got closer to his house, my anxiety kicked in. What would I be facing? Would he be alert? Would he welcome me or be irritable? I wondered about the wisdom of taking this hospice job.

The note on the front door indicated that it was unlocked. I knocked and walked inside. Slowly I climbed the stairs, wishing for more stairs. I heard a woman whisper, "She's here." The bedroom door was ajar. I was shocked to see a skeleton of a man. Although his eyes were closed, I hurriedly put on the gown, mask and gloves, hoping he didn't feel humiliated by my protective garb.

Walking into the room, I felt like a zombie. When I introduced myself, he gave a barely audible moan, never opening his eyes. I drew up the pain medication in the syringe, praying that there would be enough flesh to give the injection. He moaned again as I gently turned him on his side. "So sorry," I said, as he winced with pain. This man, not yet thirty-five years old, was actively dying. There was so little I could do for him.

I asked him if I could ease him into the chair and straighten the sheets on his bed. He didn't speak but nodded his head and opened his eyes. Could he see the compassion in my eyes above the mask? "So sorry," became my mantra each time the look of pain crossed his face. He shook his head when I asked if he wanted a sip of water. He nodded when I inquired about moistening his parched lips. I was grateful I could provide some comfort to him.

I made brief notes in his medical chart and spoke with the caregiver. His sister looked lost in grief. Without wanting an answer, she quietly asked, "How can you do this kind of work?" I smiled and touched her shoulder.

Preparing to leave, I went to my patient to say goodbye. He murmured something, and I bent down closer to hear him. His words stunned me. Where did he get the strength to utter them?

He whispered, "There must be a special place in heaven for people like you."

His name is long forgotten. His profound words will stay with me forever.

~Rosanne Trost

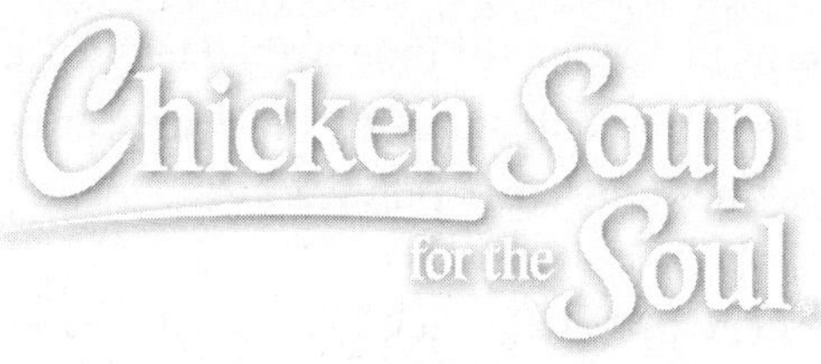

Meet Our Contributors

Alyssa Annunziato recently received her master's degree in Clinical Psychology from Vanguard University. After her yearlong battle with cancer and a diagnosis of myasthenia gravis, Alyssa hopes to encourage and inspire others by sharing her story. She is also in the process of becoming a licensed therapist.

Craig S. Baker is a freelance writer and journalist. He received his B.A. degree in Creative Writing with Honors from the University of Arizona in Tucson, where he lives with his wife and three dogs. Craig also maintains the blog "Starting From Scratch," which offers writing advice from industry professionals at CraigSBaker.com.

Judy Mae Benson received her BSN degree from the University of Phoenix in 2008 and her CNOR in 1992. She lives in Eastern Washington State with her significant other Terry and daughter Melissa. She is an operating room ANM and enjoys hiking, vintage Barbie dolls, Mariners baseball and cruising the world.

Christine Bielecki has been a registered nurse in hospice care for over fourteen years. Her interaction with the patients and their loved ones is an inspiration to her. Nursing is her vocation rather than a career. She is the proud grandmother of eight beautiful children. She plans to write a hospice book.

A writer, teacher, and editor, **Bruce Black** graduated from Columbia University and earned his MFA degree in writing from Vermont

College (now Vermont College of Fine Arts). He is the author of *Writing Yoga* (Rodmell Press), and his stories have appeared in *Cricke*t and *Cobblestone* magazines and other publications.

Barbara Brady lives in Topeka, KS with her husband of sixty years. Barbara has previously been published in Chicken Soup for the Soul books. She finds pleasure in family, friends, reading and writing.

Cassandra Brent is the pseudonym for an author, poet, playwright, and screenwriter with ten letters after her name. She's a Literary Midwife with more than two decades of teaching classes on everything from Creative Writing in an Upward Bound Program to Dramatic Technique for Fiction Writers. Her favorite color is periwinkle.

Nancy Brooks received her Nursing Diploma from Mercy St. Vincent Medical Center in Toledo Ohio and Bachelor's of Science degree in Nursing from Eastern Michigan University *magna cum laude*. She enjoys time with her family and advocates for autistic families. She's been a NICU RN for over twenty-five years in Michigan and Ohio.

Jackie Brumley received her BSN degree with Honors in 2008, MSN with Honors in 2013, and is the Unit Manager at the VA Hospital Cancer Care Center. Jackie enjoys quilting, being outdoors, reading and traveling with her husband and two sons. With a passion for writing, this is the first story she has submitted for publication.

Annettee Budzban is a Christian author, inspirational speaker, life coach and nurse living in the Chicagoland area. Her column "Christian Inspirations" is featured weekly in the *Daily Herald*, Lake County, IL. Her writings appear other places such as Guideposts books and magazines. E-mail her at annetteebudzban@aol.com.

Jill Burns lives in the mountains of West Virginia with her wonderful family. She's a retired piano teacher and performer. Jill enjoys writing, music, gardening, nature, and spending time with her grandchildren.

Elizabeth Carroll has worked as a registered nurse for over twenty-five years. She has enjoyed the fine art of giving great care combined with a life of praying for her patients. She has held the hands of one dying and has spoken words of hope to the one held captive in a coma. E-mail her at lizabethcarroll@yahoo.com.

Mary Carroll-Hackett holds an MFA from Bennington College. She is the author of *The Real Politics of Lipstick*, *Animal Soul*, *If We Could Know Our Bones*, and *The Night I Heard Everything*. She teaches at Longwood University in Virginia. She is working on a memoir.

Penelope Childers is a published author and enjoys writing inspirational true stories. She and her husband enjoy traveling and live in Central California. E-mail her at pachilders@comcast.net.

Michelle Civalier received her B.S. degree in Biomedical Engineering from Arizona State University in 2005. She has authored several other short works, including two in *Chicken Soup for the Soul: New Moms*. Her long-term goal is to find time to write something longer than 1,200 words. E-mail her at michelle_civalier@cox.net.

Mary Clary is a retired cardiology research nurse. She is currently a Volunteer RN in the hospital setting. Mary is now able to give back by fulfilling her need to take care of people.

Amanda Conley received her Bachelor of Nursing degree from LaSalle University and currently is enrolled in their nurse anesthesia program. She dedicates her story to her loving husband Kevin and beautiful eight-month-old daughter, Stella Marie. She also thanks her family for their love and support.

Lorri Danzig holds a master's degree in Jewish Studies. She teaches non-denominational programs for elders that approach aging as a journey of deepening wisdom and expanded possibilities. Her essays and poetry are published in journals and anthologies. Contact her at www.letitshinejourneys.com or e-mail lbdanzig@letitshinejourneys.com.

Doug Dascenzo received his Bachelor of Science degree in Professional Nursing from Wayne State University–Detroit in 1984. In 2000, he completed his MSN degree in Nursing Administration at Madonna University, Livonia, MI. Doug is currently attending the University of Pittsburgh where he is pursuing his DNP in Executive Leadership.

Flora Dash was raised in Eugene, OR and now resides in New York City. She enjoys spending time with her many pets, which include hamsters, parakeets, and dogs. She received her master's degree in Forest Ecology, and will soon spend three months in Poland's Białowieza Forest researching avian species.

Jill Davis lives with her husband Gary in Florida. She enjoys scrapbooking when she isn't writing.

Jo Davis has works published in many magazines and newspapers. At present she is in the process of illustrating the first book in her inspirational children's series, *The Treekin Legacy Collection*. Jo enjoys gardening, traveling, working on her farm with her horses, and camping.

Dr. Bob Dent earned his Doctorate in Nursing Practice from Texas Tech University Health Sciences Center. He has been a nurse and healthcare executive for more than twenty-five years. Bob is currently the Chief Operating Officer at Midland Memorial Hospital in Midland, TX. Bob values his family, faith and lifelong learning.

Brenda Dickie received her Registered Practical Nurse degree with Honours in 2003 at the age of forty-five. She is married with two adult sons. She works in palliative care full time in a hospital. She enjoys photography and nature.

Cassidy Doolittle graduated with her BSN degree and went on to attend writing school at the Institute of Children's Literature. She lives in Fort Worth, TX and stays home to freelance write and wrangle her two little boys. She loves strong coffee and funny friends.

Glenna Eady and her husband Alan live simply and close to the land in Paradise, CA. She works on a Cardiac Neuro unit at Feather River Hospital and is amazed that they graciously welcomed her back into acute care after a twenty-seven-year absence. God gives her strength and love for the work.

Alice Facente has been an RN for over thirty-five years, earning an MSN degree from University of Hartford in 2001. She has worked in patient education, home care, as a clinical instructor for the UCONN School of Nursing, and currently as the community education nurse at Backus Hospital in Connecticut.

Trish Featherstone is a long-divorced mother of two grown daughters. Her nursing career spans forty-two years in Quebec, Ontario, British Columbia and California. A long-time activist for animal rights, she currently lives in British Columbia with her rescue dog and one-eyed cat. "Nocturnal Poet" is her first publishing attempt.

Malinda Dunlap Fillingim lives in Leland, NC, and teaches ESL in a local community college.

Carole Fowkes is a registered nurse and began her career in Elyria, OH. She is also the author of a mystery novella and is currently working on a cozy mysteries series. She is married and lives with her husband in Dallas, TX.

Mary Gagnon received her ADN from Mott Community College, Flint, MI, in 1990 and her Bachelor's of Science in Nursing from Chamberlain College of Nursing in 2011. She is a critical care nurse at the University of Michigan Hospital and has been for the last twenty-five years. She is married, has two dogs and loves to fish.

Carol Gaido-Schmidt received her BSN from Penn State University in 1995, and her MBA from Penn State Erie, The Behrend College in 2002. She currently works in school health and is finishing the manuscript for her first novel.

Marcia Gaye wrote and directed her first stage play at age nine. Her poetry, essays and short stories have been published in various anthologies, winning multiple awards. She continues to work on a memoir and a historical western novel. Marcia is the mother of two grown children and wife to a very supportive husband.

Robyn Gerland is the author of *All These Long Years Later,* a book of short stories that may be found in both the Vancouver Island and Vancouver Library systems. She is the past editor of *The Kitchener/ Waterloo* glossy, *Hysteria*, and has been a contributor and columnist for several newspapers and magazines.

Ivani Greppi is a registered nurse and Legal Nurse Consultant. She's been married to Maciel for thirty-six years. They have two adult children, Andre and Carla, and one grandson Andre Jr. Ivani currently resides in Florida, and is writing a fiction Christian novel based on spiritual warfare and the dangers of occult practices.

Catherine Hannah Grey is a pseudonym for the writer of this story. She looks forward to the day when she can use her birth name freely because people are unafraid of her condition. Retired from human services, she now writes, volunteers, and advocates for people with DID. Catherine loves walking and cat time.

Maureen Hager is a writer, blogger and speaker. Her message of hope and healing out of brokenness is a testimony of the power of God's transforming love. She is an advocate for anti-human-trafficking. Maureen and her husband live in Western North Carolina. They have two grown daughters. Learn more at www.MaureenHager.com.

Mary Lynn Harrison has a BSN from the University of Michigan. She has worked as a nurse in Pediatric and Neonatal ICUs, in a freestanding Birth Center, as clinical faculty, and is currently a school nurse in a school that serves physically impaired students. Her latest favorite hobby is her grandchildren.

Colleen Haynes completed an MA degree at fifty-something through Royal Roads University, then retired from nursing, having worked in emergency, home care, psych/mental health, and academia. She lives in Edmonton, Canada with her husband Michael and works as a freelance writer, editor, and recipe blogger. E-mail her at cls03@shaw.ca.

Marijo Herndon currently lives in New York with her husband Dave and two rescue cats, Lucy and Ethel. Marijo's stories, ranging from humor to inspiration, appear in numerous books and publications.

Jacqueline Hickey lives with her husband in beautiful Rockport, MS, where she enjoys running, writing and spending time with her family.

Sandra Hickman is a nonfiction writer, poet, and songwriter from Western Australia. She enjoys writing about her missionary work in Africa, India and China. A Bible School graduate, Sandra now serves in Church leadership. Her book, *The Letter*, will be published in 2015. E-mail her at sandrevival@yahoo.com.au.

Dr. Sharon T. Hinton, **DMIN**, **RN-BC**, **MSN** is a specialist for the International Parish Nurse Resource Center, Executive Director of Rural Nurse Resource, and a national speaker and seminar leader. She lives in rural Texas with a menagerie of pets including cows and wildlife. Writing is her favorite pastime!

Ms. Hopkins received her ADN and BSN from Midway College. She is also a patented inventor. She lives in Kentucky with her husband, two sons and daughter-in-law. She has practiced nursing for the past thirty-five years and enjoys writing, making crafts and attending church.

Jennie Ivey lives in Tennessee. She is the author of various works of fiction and nonfiction, including several stories in the Chicken Soup for the Soul collection. Learn more at jennieivey.com.

Phyllis Jardine, a retired nurse and grandmother, writes from the Annapolis Valley, Nova Scotia, where she lives with her husband Bud. Her inspirational essays and poems have been widely published and heard on national radio. This is Phyllis's fourth story in the Chicken Soup for the Soul series.

Kathleen Jones worked as a pediatric nurse before embarking on her present career as a freelance writer. She has been published in professional nursing magazines, as a contributor to the *IV Drug Handbook* by McGraw-Hill, and as a writer for children's educational publishers. Currently she is writing for Tango and Tilly Press.

Mariah Julio has published stories and articles in *Faith, Hope and Fiction*, *This I Believe*, *Patchwork Path: Friendship Star*, *Flair* magazine and newspapers. She has completed writing courses offered by Western Kentucky University. A retired nurse, Mariah enjoys travel, writing, painting and futile attempts to outwit her cat.

Eva Juliuson remarried after her first husband's death. She and Dwight have seven children along with their spouses, twelve grandchildren and a great grandchild. Eva loves teaching preschool children, writing, landscaping and the adventure of living each day with the Lord!

Molly K. is a registered nurse in the Washington, DC metro area where she lives with her husband and her dog. She is passionate about oncology and an advocate for continued research into new cancer treatments. Molly is currently studying to become a Family Nurse Practitioner.

Pallavi Kamat is a doctor by profession and a writer by passion. She has managed to take baby steps into the writing world, with whatever time she can squeeze out of her hectic schedule. She hopes her dream of writing a novel will be fulfilled in the foreseeable future.

Alioune Kotey received his associate's degree in Nursing from Norwalk Community College and went on to complete his bachelor's degree in Nursing from Sacred Heart University. He is married, enjoys traveling and is a published professional photographer, following in the footsteps of his father, who was an awarding-winning amateur photographer.

Delores Liesner's motto, putting hands and feet to our faith, is revealed in the true stories in her book titled *Be The Miracle!* (2015 Elk Lake Publishing). She aims for her writing to benefit children. Learn more at deloresliesner.com.

Emily Linegar is a student at Brandon University. She hopes to become a teacher one day, but will keep writing on the side.

Diana Lynn is a small business owner and a freelance writer in Washington State. She has been a Chicken Soup for the Soul contributor for five years. Her interests are reading, running, writing, and dancing. She dedicates this story to her mother, who was a nurse for thirty-five years.

Nancy Mapes received her Bachelor of Science degree in Nursing from the University of Texas at Arlington. She has two grown children and two grandchildren. Of course, she loves to spend any spare time with her grandchildren. She also loves reading. This is her first publication.

Donna Mason received her nursing degree in 1977 from Cochise College in Arizona. She still continues to practice nursing in the rural Southwest. Donna has been married for thirty-seven years, has two daughters and two grandsons. She enjoys travel, fishing, rockhounding, reading and spending time with her family.

Bette Haywood Matero is a retired childcare professional and children's ministry director. Writing has always been her passion and after moving to Arizona with her husband, she has finally found the time to follow that passion. She is the mother of three wonderful adult children; and has one much loved granddaughter.

Kathy McGovern is a well-known speaker and writer in the Denver area, where she lives blissfully with her wonderful husband Ben Lager. She writes a weekly scripture column for parish bulletins. Subscribe by visiting www.thestoryandyou.com.

Diana M. Millikan was born in England and grew up during the Second World War, where she lost her home to bombing. She is a retired nurse and lives with her husband and pets on a small island in Puget Sound. She enjoys her grandchildren, gardening and photography.

Marya Morin is a freelance writer. Her stories have appeared in publications such as *Woman's World* and Hallmark. Marya also penned a weekly humorous column for an online newsletter, and writes custom poetry on request. She lives in the country with her husband. E-mail her at Akushla514@hotmail.com.

Andy Myers is a full-time psychic medium, best-selling author, and inspirational speaker based out of Omaha, NE. He's featured on radio stations nationwide and conducts sold-out events across the country. Andy holds a bachelor's degree in Social Work and enjoys watching soccer with his wife and one-year-old daughter.

Linda Newton is an Empowerment Educator, and the author of *12 Ways to Turn Your Pain Into Praise*. She speaks all over the country, and currently hosts a popular vlog with her husband, "Answers from Mom and Dad," on YouTube at www.youtube.com/channel/UCWi1JpTWiT32ZiGwhb971hQ and www.facebook.com/answersfrommomanddad.

Phyllis Nordstrom spent most of her career working in the business and church worlds as she assisted her husband in pastoring. They are the parents of four children, and grandparents to twelve grandchildren and one great-grandchild. She is a breast cancer survivor. Writing now joins teaching, traveling, reading, and swimming as hobbies.

Judy Pencek attended the Robert Packer Hospital's School of Nursing and has enjoyed caring for patients since graduating in 1977. She is the proud mother of three daughters and grandma to eight grandchildren. Judy has published many devotionals and is preparing to publish her first book of nursing stories.

Connie Kaseweter Pullen received her Bachelor of Arts degree, *cum laude*, from the University of Portland in 2006, with a double major in Psychology and Sociology. Connie enjoys running, writing and photography. The proud mother of five children and grandmother of several grandchildren recently had four stories published in Hallmark books.

Jennifer Quasha is a freelance writer and editor who has published over forty books for adults and children. She loves writing for Chicken Soup for the Soul and has been published in over twenty Chicken Soup for the Soul books. Learn more at jenniferquasha.com.

Jeff Radford received his Bachelor's of Science degree in Nursing from Old Dominion University, Master's of Business Administration degree from Baker College, and Doctor of Strategic Leadership degree from Regent University. His passion is to exhibit merciful leadership and serve others. He is dedicated to his church and family.

Amy Rivers was a SANE Director for two years. She received her master's degree with concentrations in Psychology and Political Science in 2014. She lives with her fiancé and two children in Colorado. Amy enjoys writing, singing and political activism. She plans to continue her work in violence prevention.

Tracy Rose-Tynes, RN, received her degree from Northeastern University. Her expertise is in Adolescent Medicine. She works at a school-based health center in Cambridge, MA. Tracy is also a singer-songwriter. She performs regularly at school for her students, at the hospital for special events and at local jazz clubs.

Mark Rosolowski is a Navy veteran, and has worked as a corpsman, paramedic, and a security and safety supervisor in a hospital. Mark is married to Jeanette, who is a registered nurse. Mark would like to dedicate his story to all dialysis nurses. E-mail him at rpolishprince@aol.com.

Ceil Ryan is a wife, nurse, mom and nana living in the Midwest. After over twenty years, she hung up her nurse's cap to write full-time. Her passion is sharing personal stories with an emphasis on faith and encouragement. Read more from Ceil at www.ceilryan.com, and follow her on facebook.com/surroundedbythespirit.

Beth Saadati is currently teaching high school writing classes, homeschooling her son and daughter, and drafting two narrative nonfiction books. In the aftermath of her beloved firstborn's suicide, she shares a message of hope and continues to invest her heart into the lives of teens. E-mail her at bethsaadati@gmail.com.

Thom Schwarz has been a hospice and palliative care nurse for seven years. Prior to that he was the editorial director of the *American Journal of Nursing*. He has been writing since he could hold a pencil. He almost has it mastered.

Bev Schwind graduated from Nursing in 1972 and was named Student Nurse of the Year. She and her husband Jim, of sixty-two years, have four children (three are nurses) and sixteen grandchildren. Bev writes devotionals on assignment and has authored five books. In the Senior Olympics she won National medals in softball, basketball and tennis.

Leanne Sells has been a nurse for twenty-three years, primarily in Women's Health and Pediatrics. She is currently an L&D nurse manager and an advocate for evidence-based practice and the evolution of nursing practice with today's technology. She is a wife, mother of three, and an avid sports fan.

Debbie Sistare has a B.S. degree in Nursing and a master's degree in Religious Psychology. Her thirty-year nursing career included pediatric nursing, flight nursing, nursing instructor and hospital supervisor. She enjoys her large family, reading, writing, needlepoint and her three dogs.

Alisa Smith worked as an ICU nurse after graduating from Duke University and now lives in Chapel Hill, NC, surrounded by her four children and two grandchildren.

Linda Smith was an operating room registered nurse for thirty-eight years. Following a 2007 early retirement she began hosting a local television talk show, *Lynchburg Live*, self-published a volume of poetry and prose and is a freelance author. She is a seven-year breast cancer survivor, a wife and stepmom who speaks at breast cancer seminars.

Cheryll Snow has been a registered nurse for twenty-five years. Her patients have taught her much about life and loss. She is a frequent contributor to the Chicken Soup for the Soul series. She is currently seeking representation for her inspirational fiction novel, titled *Sea Horses*.

Brenda Stiverson became a registered nurse in 1994, fulfilling her lifelong dream. She has three children and six grandchildren and loves her job managing an orthopedic unit in Oklahoma. Brenda enjoys reading, movies, and traveling, but her favorite pastime is spending time with her family. E-mail her at brennie@cox.net.

Sharon Stoika-Smay is married and lives with her family and two dogs in a small coal-mining town in Western Pennsylvania. She also has a home in St Petersburg, FL. She has been a nurse for nearly thirty-eight years. Her hobbies include reading, writing, calligraphy, Zentangle, and pysanky Ukrainian egg art.

Kathy Stringham has worked in a variety of nursing departments throughout her career, in addition to working as an entrepreneur for fifteen years. She is currently a hospice manager in Southeastern Michigan. She lives with her husband and has two grown children. Kathy enjoys Pilates, yoga, creative cooking, and the outdoors.

Gladys Swedak started writing seriously in 2000 with a bi-weekly contest she didn't win. She has written and self-published two novels: *The Wild Ones*, about training wild horses without their knowledge, and *White Medicine Woman*, about a young woman adopted by a medicine woman of an Indian tribe.

Annette Tersigni, RN, is a former Hollywood actor and cover girl turned nurse, author, and inspirational speaker. She is the founder of YogaNursing®, a new movement in nursing and yoga. Annette is a successful nurse entrepreneur who has motivated thousands of people to lead healthier and more spiritual lives.

Terrie Todd has published seven previous stories in the Chicken Soup for the Soul series, two plays with Eldridge Plays & Musicals, and writes a weekly faith and humor column for the *Central Plains Herald Leader*. In 2010, she served on the editorial advisory board for *Chicken Soup for the Soul: O Canada*. She lives in Manitoba.

Rosanne Trost is a retired registered nurse living in Houston, TX. She spent most of her career in oncology nursing. Since retirement, she has developed a passion for creative writing.

Kosuke Vasquez earned his B.A. degree in Communication from the University of Hawaii in 1983. He retired in 2008, after a thirty-seven-year career in federal government. His wife of thirty-five years, a registered nurse, passed away in 2014. He has two grown children and lives in Alexandria, VA. E-mail him at kv5x5@cox.net.

Helen Wilder, a former kindergarten/first grade teacher in southeastern Kentucky, is married with one daughter, a son-in-law, and a grandpuppy, Paco. She enjoys teaching young children, reading, scrapbooking, storytelling, and writing inspirational articles. She enjoys volunteering with Friends of the Library.

Kimberly Yates is a writer and online community moderator. She and her husband live in Oklahoma, where she considers herself a professional spoiler of her nieces, nephews and the crazy animals who share her home. She is working on a book of humorous essays.

Lynn Zoll has a Bachelor of Science degree in Nursing, and is a registered nurse. Currently she is a certified School Nurse and works at West Deptford High School. In her off time she works for Mainstage Center for the Arts, a non-profit performing arts center.

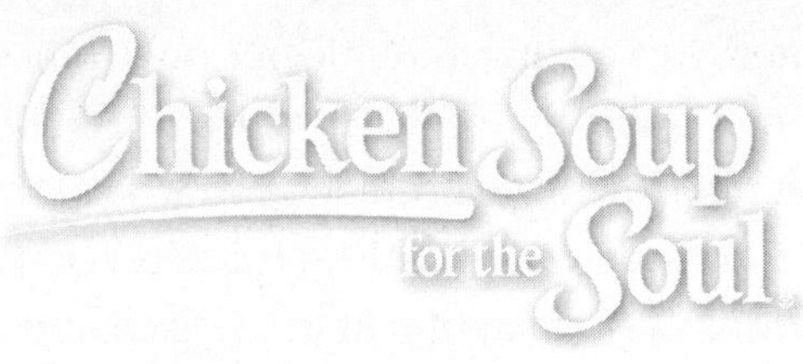

Meet Amy Newmark

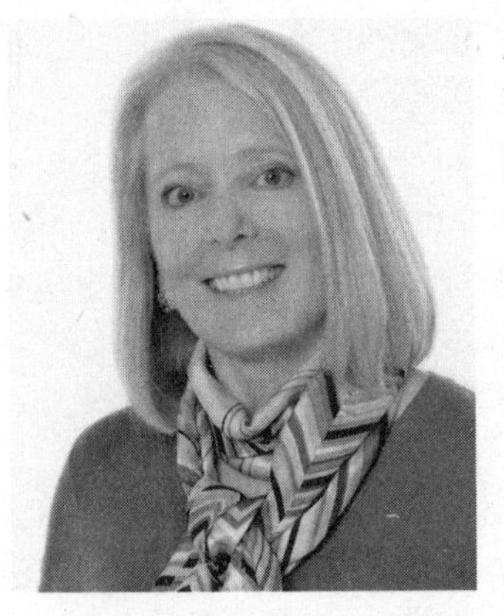

Amy Newmark was a writer, speaker, Wall Street analyst and business executive in the worlds of finance and telecommunications for thirty years. Today she is publisher, editor-in-chief and coauthor of the Chicken Soup for the Soul book series. By curating and editing inspirational true stories from ordinary people who have had extraordinary experiences, Amy has kept the twenty-two-year-old Chicken Soup for the Soul brand fresh and relevant, and still part of the social zeitgeist.

Amy graduated *magna cum laude* from Harvard University where she majored in Portuguese and minored in French. She wrote her thesis about popular, spoken-word poetry in Brazil, which involved traveling throughout Brazil and meeting with poets and writers to collect their stories. She is delighted to have come full circle in her writing career — from collecting poetry "from the people" in Brazil as a twenty-year-old to, three decades later, collecting stories and poems "from the people" for Chicken Soup for the Soul.

Amy has a national syndicated newspaper column and is a frequent radio and TV guest, passing along the real-life lessons and useful tips she has picked up from reading and editing thousands of Chicken Soup for the Soul stories.

She and her husband are the proud parents of four grown children and in her limited spare time, Amy enjoys visiting them, hiking, and reading books that she did not have to edit.

Follow her on Twitter @amynewmark and @chickensoupsoul.

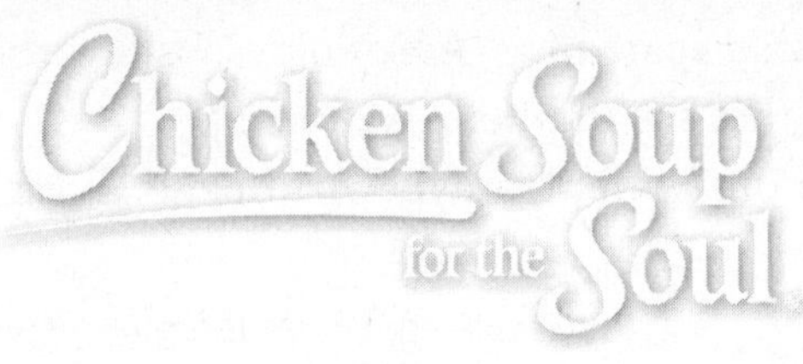

Meet LeAnn Thieman

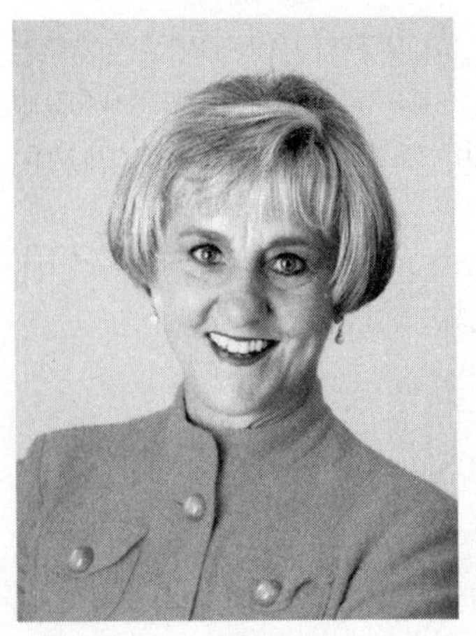

LeAnn's story of being "accidentally" caught up in the Vietnam Orphan Airlift in 1975 engages and inspires people as they learn her tools for coping in the war zones of their everyday lives. An ordinary person, she struggled through extraordinary circumstances and found the courage to succeed during her daring adventure of helping to rescue 300 babies as Saigon was falling to the Communists. LeAnn's penetrating conversations and expertise have been featured around the globe on BBC, NPR, PBS, FOX News, *Newsweek* magazine's "Voices of the Century" issue, and countless radio and TV programs.

LeAnn's fifteen books have inspired, motivated, and changed the lives of millions of readers. It began with "This Must Be My Brother," her incredible "Operation Babylift" story. After it was featured in *Chicken Soup for the Mother's Soul*, LeAnn became one of Chicken Soup's most prolific writers.

Her devotion to thirty years of nursing made her the ideal co-author of *Chicken Soup for the Nurse's Soul*, which hit the New York Times Bestseller list! She went on to co-author *Chicken Soup for the Nurse's Soul, Second Dose*; *Chicken Soup for the Christian Woman's Soul*; *Chicken Soup for the Caregiver's Soul*; *Chicken Soup for the Father and Daughter Soul*; *Chicken Soup for the Grandma's Soul*; *Chicken Soup for the Mother and Son Soul*; *Chicken Soup for the Christian Soul 2*; *Chicken*

Soup for the Adopted Soul (re-released as Chicken Soup for the Soul: The Joy of Adoption); *Chicken Soup for the Soul: Living Catholic Faith*; *Chicken Soup for the Soul: A Book of Miracles* and *Chicken Soup for the Soul: Answered Prayers.*

Her latest book, *SelfCare for HealthCare™*, *Your Guide to Physical, Mental and Spiritual Health*, is a dynamic component of her transformational SelfCare for HealthCare initiative.

LeAnn is among fewer than ten percent of expert speakers worldwide to have earned the Certified Speaking Professional designation and in August 2008 she was inducted into the National Speakers Association's Speaker Hall of Fame, further motivating people to say, "I'm going to live my life differently after hearing you today."

She and Mark, her husband of forty-five years, reside in Colorado.

For more information about LeAnn's books and products or to schedule her for a presentation or her SelfCare for HealthCare™ program, please contact her at:

LeAnn Thieman, CSP, CPAE
6600 Thompson Drive
Fort Collins, CO 80526
1-970-223-1574
www.LeAnnThieman.com
LeAnn@LeAnnThieman.com

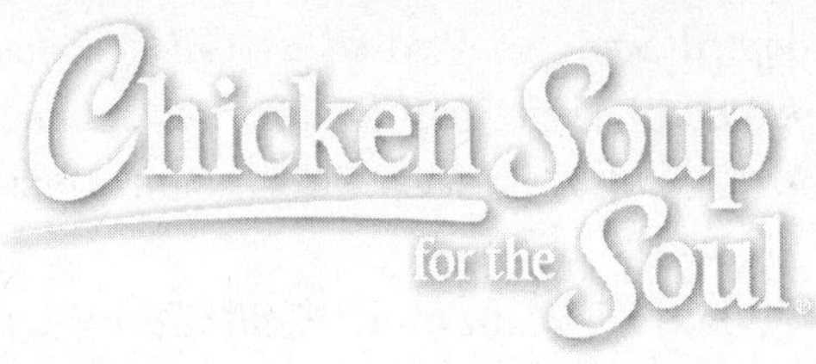

Thank You

We owe huge thanks to all of our contributors. We know that you poured your hearts and souls into the thousands of stories that you shared with us. We appreciate your willingness to open up your lives to other nurses and healthcare professionals and share your own experiences, no matter how personal. We could only publish a small percentage of the stories that were submitted, but we read every single one and even the ones that do not appear in the book had an influence on us and on the final manuscript.

We are so grateful to Ronelle Frankel, whose editorial assistance provided immense efficiency and joy to this project. And we want to deliver a special thanks to LeAnn's team members Jaejin Kim and Katie Hanna, who kept her speaking business thriving while she devoted time and attention to this book, furthering her mission to nurture nurses.

Assistant publisher D'ette Corona did her normal masterful job working with us and all the story contributors on edits, and editors Barbara LoMonaco, Marti Davidson Sichel, and Kristiana Pastir helped proofread the final layout. We are grateful for the very special Chicken Soup for the Soul publishing team.

~Amy Newmark and LeAnn Thieman

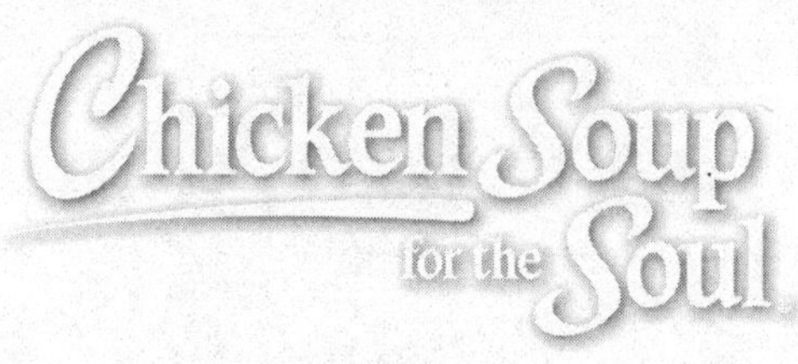

Sharing Happiness, Inspiration, and Wellness

Real people sharing real stories, every day, all over the world. In 2007, *USA Today* named *Chicken Soup for the Soul* one of the five most memorable books in the last quarter-century. With over 100 million books sold to date in the U.S. and Canada alone, more than 200 titles in print, and translations into more than forty languages, "chicken soup for the soul" is one of the world's best-known phrases.

Today, twenty-two years after we first began sharing happiness, inspiration and wellness through our books, we continue to delight our readers with new titles, but have also evolved beyond the bookstore, with super premium pet food, a line of high quality food to bring people together for healthy meals, and a variety of licensed products and digital offerings, all inspired by stories. Chicken Soup for the Soul has recently expanded into visual storytelling through movies and television. Chicken Soup for the Soul is "changing the world one story at a time®." Thanks for reading!

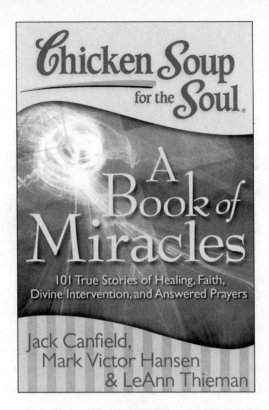

Everyone loves a good miracle story, and this book provides 101 true stories of healing, divine intervention, and answered prayers. These amazing, personal stories prove that God is alive and active in the world today, working miracles on our behalf. The incredible accounts show His love and involvement in our lives. This book of miracles will encourage, uplift, and recharge the faith of all Christian readers

978-1-935096-51-1

Faith, hope and miracles

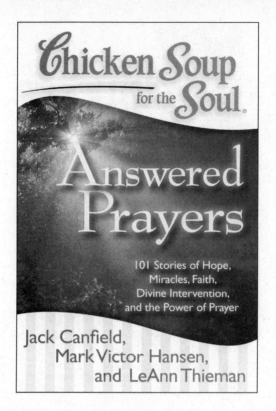

We all need help from time to time, and these 101 true stories about the power of prayer show a higher power at work in our lives. Regular people share their personal stories of God's Divine intervention, healing power, and communication. Evidence of His love and involvement in our lives will encourage, uplift, and recharge the faith of all readers.

978-1-935096-76-4

to restore your soul

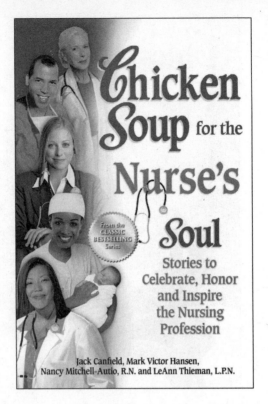

The national bestseller that inspired a generation of nurses! You'll laugh and cry along with these true stories from all types of nurses—about the patients who affected them most deeply, their personal ups and downs as nurses, their funniest moments, their most heartwarming experiences. And there are lots of great tips from the people who make an important difference in the lives of patients and their families.

978-1-62361-102-6

More inspiration
& relaxation

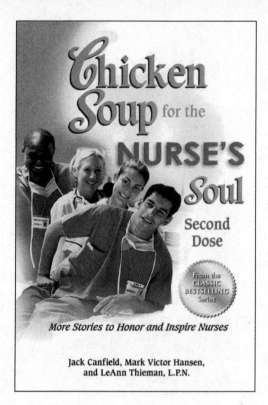

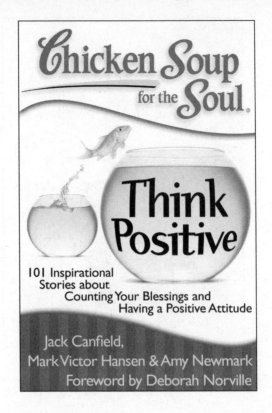

Every cloud has a silver lining. You will be inspired by these 101 real-life stories from people just like you, about taking a positive attitude to the ups and downs of life, and remembering to be grateful and count their blessings. These inspirational stories of hope, optimism, and faith will encourage you to stay positive during challenging times and in your everyday life.

978-1-935096-56-6

Positive thinking and

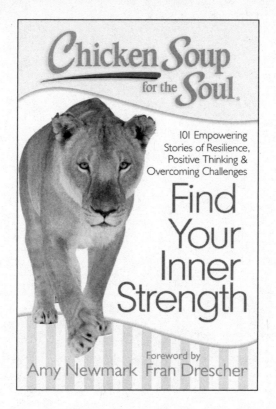

We're all stronger than we think, and we often discover our inner strength and resilience when a problem arises. The 101 empowering and uplifting stories in this collection by people who have overcome challenges, solved problems, or changed their lives will help you find your own inner strength, resilience, and remind you to think positive, count your blessings, and use the power that you have within you.

978-1-61159-939-8

models of resilience